Engaging Communities for Improving Mothers' and Children's Health

Reviewing the Evidence of Effectiveness in Resource-Constrained Settings

Edited by
Henry B Perry

Published in the United Kingdom by JoGH.

JoGH is an imprint of the Edinburgh University Global Health Society.

Edinburgh University Global Health Society
Teviot Place, Edinburgh EH8 9AG
Scotland, United Kingdom

Printed in Croatia by LaserPLUS, Ltd.

ISBN-13: 978-0-9933638-5-6

Front cover photocredit:

Engaging Communities for Improving Mothers' and Children's Health

Reviewing the Evidence of Effectiveness in Resource-Constrained Settings

Edited by

Henry B Perry

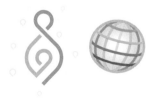

2017

Pioneers in community-based primary health care made this book possible. So, above all, we want to remember people who, beginning in the mid-20th century, had a vision for alternative approaches that made it possible to implement programs that engaged communities to improve the health of mothers and children using scientific evidence from medicine and public health that could be applied in settings where there was a shortage of highly trained medical personnel and health facilities. In this regard, four such pioneers – Dr. Carl Taylor, Dr. John Wyon, and Drs. Warren and Gretchen Berggren – provided me with inspiration, mentorship and friendship which have guided my contributions to this work.

More than 150 people contributed to the collection and analysis of the information contained in this book, and I am grateful to all of them, most of whom did this on a voluntary basis. Small grants were provided along the way to cover unavoidable expenses. I am grateful to the World Health Organization, UNICEF, the World Bank, the United States Agency for International Development, the American Public Health Association, and Future Generations for their support for this project, which took more than a decade to complete.

Henry B Perry, September 2017

Contents

PREFACE

Community–based primary health care: a core strategy for achieving sustainable development goals for health

Zulfiqar A Bhutta

Centre for Global Child Health, The Hospital for Sick Children, Toronto, Canada

A major barrier to the achievement of Millennium Development Goals (MDGs) for reducing maternal and child mortality by three quarters and two–thirds respectively, related to lack of access to care by millions living in abject poverty in rural populations and urban slums [1]. Notwithstanding the challenges, with extraordinary efforts by countries and development partners in the MDG era, child mortality has seen a remarkable decline. Under–five deaths decreased from 12.7 million in 1990 to 5.8 million in 2015 with an increase in the annual rate of under–five mortality reduction from 1.8% over the period 1990–2000 to 3.9% over 2000–2015. However, corresponding progress in reducing neonatal mortality has been less substantial, and the approximate 2.6 million neonates who die every year account for nearly half of all under–five deaths. The annual rate of decrease of neonatal mortality stands at 2.9%, as compared to 4.9% for the 1–59 month age group over this period [2,3].

These gains in global maternal and child health and survival are by no means equal and wide global disparities persist. Sub–Saharan Africa continues to have the highest under–five mortality rate among all regions, with 83 deaths per 1000 live births annually. Although Millennium Development Goal 4 was achieved in some high–mortality countries in Sub–Saharan Africa and South Asia, there are still 58 low– and middle–income countries (LMICs) who are still to reach this target. Barriers to access and equitable care are related to poverty and compounded by lack of trained human resources for health and poorly functional health systems.

In 2015, the world transitioned from the MDGs to the Sustainable Development Goals (SDGs). Although the maternal, neonatal, child and adolescent health issues remain central, the SDGs are all encompassing and the health goal (SDG3) will require close linkages with other contributing SDGs. Although lack of skilled birth attendants and qualified health workers is a large part of the problem, poor health outcomes also related to complex issues such as maternal empowerment, sociocultural taboos, and care–seeking practices and behaviors during pregnancy and child–birth [4]. Given the clustering of maternal and newborn burden of disease in rural settings and among the urban poor we need strategies for promoting community demand as well as appropriate outreach through community health workers and volunteers.

The global evidence base for strategies and interventions for newborn care in community settings has substantially improved, with a range of interventions that can be potentially packaged for delivery at different times during pregnancy, childbirth, and after birth, through various health–care providers, especially community health workers (CHWs). These CHWs were tasked with improving maternal and child health outcomes in a range of research settings and shown to be effective [5]. A fundamental question is whether such concerted interventions especially promotion of behavior–change interventions can be applied in real health systems with busy schedules of health workers and competing priorities. A recent collation of evidence from national programs suggests that this strategy can be effective [6]. Studies evaluating women's groups, frequently supported by community volunteers show consistent benefits on improved maternal and newborn outcomes [7]. These studies also provide strong evidence that community–based strategies for preventive newborn care substantially improve domiciliary practices, care–seeking patterns, and newborn survival. The case for the scaling–up of strategies for preventive newborn care in community settings with a range of participatory approaches is thus very strong.

Much of the global evidence for community based strategies for care has been collated in systematic reviews with an undue reliance on randomized controlled trials [8]. This supplement collates a vast amount of information from community–based studies of strategies and programs to improve maternal and child health and immunization outcomes, and enhances the evidence in several ways. Dr Perry and colleagues painstakingly collected and reviewed a large body of information from almost 700 reports and studies exploring various aspects of the cumulative experience of community based primary health care globally [9]. The studies comprise of a vast amount of information and while systematic meta–analyses were not performed, the narrative reports demonstrate the effectiveness of various approaches undertaken in disparate geographies and socio–economic settings. These findings are consonant with the findings from a review of community based approaches for primary health care almost a decade ago [10] and the recent evidence synthesis undertaken by the Disease Control Priorities project.

As we move toward accelerating action for achieving the SDGs, the role of community based platforms will become more important. These strategies are needed to ensure that several of the key themes of the SDGs such as reducing inequities and reaching marginalized populations, are achieved within the next 15 years. Some 40 years following the Alma Ata declaration of "health for all", this might yet become a reality.

References

1 Victora CG, Requejo JH, Barros AJ, Berman P, Bhutta Z, Boerma T, et al. Countdown to 2015: a decade of tracking progress for maternal, newborn, and child survival. Lancet. 2016;387:2049-59. Medline:26477328 doi:10.1016/S0140-6736(15)00519-X<

2 GBD 2015 Maternal Mortality Collaborators. Global, regional, and national levels of maternal mortality, 1990-2015: a systematic analysis for the Global Burden of Disease Study 2015. Lancet. 2016;388:1775-812. Medline:27733286 doi:10.1016/S0140-6736(16)31470-2

3 GBD 2015 Mortality and Causes of Death Collaborators. Global, regional, and national life expectancy, all-cause mortality, and cause-specific mortality for 249 causes of death, 1980-2015: a systematic analysis for the Global Burden of Disease Study 2015. Lancet. 2016;388:1459-544. Medline:27733281 doi:10.1016/S0140-6736(16)31012-1

4 Bhutta ZA, Black RE. Global maternal, newborn, and child health–so near and yet so far. N Engl J Med. 2013;369:2226-35. Medline:24304052 doi:10.1056/NEJMra1111853

5 Lassi ZS, Kumar R, Bhutta ZA. Community-Based Care to Improve Maternal, Newborn, and Child Health. In: Black RE, Laxminarayan R, Temmerman M, Walker N, editors. Reproductive, Maternal, Newborn, and Child Health: Disease Control Priorities, Third Edition (Volume 2). Washington, DC: The International Bank for Reconstruction and Development/The World Bank; 2016.

6 Bhutta ZA, Lassi ZS, Pariyo GLH. Global experience of community health workers for delivery of health related Millennium Development Goals: a systematic review, country case studies, and recommendations for integration into national health systems. Geneva: WHO/Global Health Workforce Alliance, 2010.

7 Prost A, Colbourn T, Seward N, Azad K, Coomarasamy A, Copas A, et al. Women's groups practising participatory learning and action to improve maternal and newborn health in low-resource settings: a systematic review and meta-analysis. Lancet. 2013;381:1736-46. Medline:23683640 doi:10.1016/S0140-6736(13)60685-6

8 Lassi ZS, Bhutta ZA. Community-based intervention packages for reducing maternal and neonatal morbidity and mortality and improving neonatal outcomes. Cochrane Database Syst Rev. 2015;3:CD007754. Medline:25803792

9 Perry H, Rassekh BM, Gupta S, Wilhelm J, Freeman P. A comprehensive review of the evidence regarding the evidence of the effectiveness of community-based primary health care in improving maternal, newborn and child health. 1: rationale, methods and database description. J Glob Health. 2017;1:010901.

10 Bhutta ZA, Ali S, Cousens S, Ali TM, Haider BA, Rizvi A, et al. Alma-Ata: Rebirth and Revision 6 Interventions to address maternal, newborn, and child survival: what difference can integrated primary health care strategies make? Lancet. 2008;372:972-89. Medline:18790320 doi:10.1016/S0140-6736(08)61407-5

Acknowledgement: originally published as: Zulfiqar A Bhutta: Community–based primary health care: a core strategy for achieving sustainable development goals for health. Reprinted with permission from Edinburgh University Global Health Society under Creative Commons Attribution Licence (Journal of Global Health 2017; 010101).

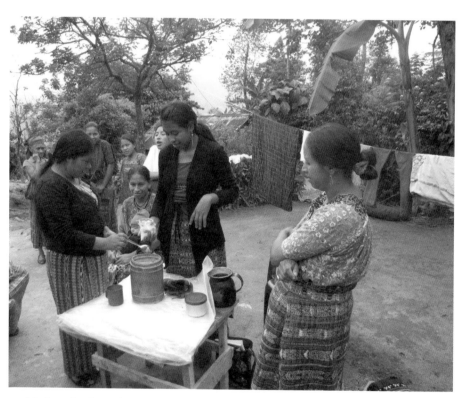

Mothers in the isolated rural mountains of Guatemala learning together how to prepare oral rehydration solution for treatment of childhood diarrhea

Photocredit: Henry Perry (used with permission).

Comprehensive review of the evidence regarding the effectiveness of community–based primary health care in improving maternal, neonatal and child health: 1. rationale, methods and database description

Henry B Perry[1], Bahie M Rassekh[2], Sundeep Gupta[3],
Jess Wilhelm[1], Paul A Freeman[4,5]

[1] Department of International Health, Johns Hopkins Bloomberg School of Public Health, Baltimore, Maryland, USA
[2] The World Bank, Washington DC, USA
[3] Medical Epidemiologist, Lusaka, Zambia
[4] Independent consultant, Seattle, Washington, USA
[5] Department of Global Health, University of Washington, Seattle, Washington, USA

Background Community–based primary health care (CBPHC) is an approach used by health programs to extend preventive and curative health services beyond health facilities into communities and even down to households. Evidence of the effectiveness of CBPHC in improving maternal, neonatal and child health (MNCH) has been summarized by others, but our review gives gives particular attention to not only the effectiveness of specific interventions but also their delivery strategies at the community level along with their equity effects. This is the first article in a series that summarizes and analyzes the assessments of programs, projects, and research studies (referred to collectively as projects) that used CBPHC to improve MNCH in low– and middle–income countries. The review addresses the following questions: (1) What kinds of projects were implemented? (2) What were the outcomes of these projects? (3) What kinds of implementation strategies were used? (4) What are the implications of these findings?

Methods 12 166 reports were identified through a search of articles in the National Library of Medicine database (PubMed). In addition, reports in the gray literature (available online but not published in a peer–reviewed journal) were also reviewed. Reports that describe the implementation of one or more community–based interventions or an integrated project in which an assessment of the effectiveness of the project was carried out qualified for inclusion in the review. Outcome measures that qualified for inclusion in the review were population–based indicators that defined some aspect of health status: changes in population coverage of evidence–based interventions or changes in serious morbidity, in nutritional status, or in mortality.

Results 700 assessments qualified for inclusion in the review. Two independent reviewers completed a data extraction form for each assessment. A third reviewer compared the two data extraction forms and resolved any differences. The maternal interventions assessed concerned education about warning signs of pregnancy and safe delivery; promotion and/or provision of antenatal care; promotion and/or provision of safe delivery by a trained birth attendant, screening and treatment for HIV infection and other maternal infections; family planning, and; HIV prevention and treatment. The neonatal and child health interventions that were assessed concerned promotion or provision of good nutrition and immunizations; promotion of healthy household behaviors and appropriate utilization of health services, diagnosis and treatment of acute neonatal and child illness; and provision and/or promotion of safe water, sanitation and hygiene. Two–thirds of assessments (63.0%) were for projects implementing three or fewer interventions in relatively small populations for relatively brief periods; half of the assessments involved fewer than 5000 women or children, and 62.9% of the assessments were for projects lasting less than 3 years. One–quarter (26.6%) of the projects were from three countries in South Asia: India, Bangladesh and Nepal. The number of reports has grown markedly during the past decade. A small number of funders supported most of the assessments, led by the United States Agency for International Development. The reviewers judged the methodology for 90% of the assessments to be adequate.

Conclusions The evidence regarding the effectiveness of community–based interventions to improve the health of mothers, neonates, and children younger than 5 years of age is growing rapidly. The database created for this review serves as the basis for a series of articles that follow this one on the effectiveness of CBPHC in improving MNCH published in the Journal of Global Health. These findings, guide this review, that are included as the last paper in this series, will help to provide the rationale for building stronger community–based platforms for delivering evidence–based interventions in high–mortality, resource–constrained settings.

The evidence that community–based interventions can improve maternal, neonatal and child health (MNCH) has been steadily growing over the past several decades [1–3]. Nonetheless, community–based primary health care (CBPHC) as an approach for engaging communities and delivering health interventions to communities and even down to each household remains an underdeveloped component of health systems in most resource–constrained settings. Except for immunizations and vitamin A supplementation, population coverage levels of evidence–based MNCH interventions in the countries with 97% of the world's maternal, neonatal and child deaths remains around 50% or less [4]. The evidence regarding the effectiveness of individual interventions provided at the community level continues to grow. We now stand in a moment of time in which the era of the United Nations' Millennium Development Goals has ended (2000–2015) and the era of the Sustainable

Development Goals has begun (2015–2030). Thus, now is an opportune time to take stock of the evidence regarding the effectiveness of community–based approaches in improving MNCH and the approaches that have been used to achieve effectiveness.

Even though major gains have been made around the world in reducing maternal, neonatal, and child mortality (MNCH), 8.8 million maternal deaths, stillbirths, neonatal deaths, and deaths of children 1–59 months of age occur each year, mostly from readily preventable or treatable conditions [5]. Only four of the 75 countries with 97% of the world's maternal, perinatal, neonatal and child deaths were able to achieve both Millennium Development Goal (MDG) 4 (which called for a two–thirds reduction in under–5 mortality by the year 2015 compared to 1990 levels) and MDG 5 (which called for a three–quarters reduction of maternal mortality) [6]. One of the important reasons for this disappointing result was the failure to implement and scale up evidence–based community–based interventions.

To date, there has been limited attention given to systematically accumulating and analyzing the broad range of evidence regarding the effectiveness of CBPHC in improving MNCH, although excellent summaries of portions of this evidence do exist [1–3,7–17]. In addition, there appears to be a rebirth of global primary health care more generally, especially in light of the upcoming 40th anniversary of the signing of the Declaration of Alma–Ata at the International Conference on Primary Health Care at Alma–Ata, Kazakhstan in 1978, sponsored by the World Health Organization and UNICEF [18]. This article is the first of a series that highlights the findings of a comprehensive review and analysis of this evidence in low– and middle–income countries (LMICs).

The context

The global primary health care movement began in the 1960s following the recognition that hospitals were not improving the health of the populations they were serving. At that time, a series of surveys of populations served by hospital–oriented Christian medical mission programs around the world demonstrated that the people who had easy access to and used the hospital regularly were no healthier than people who did not [19]. This led to the formation of the Christian Medical Commission (CMC) of the World Council of Churches, which provided a framework and a forum for new thinking about how programs can best improve the health of people in high–mortality, resource–constrained settings. In the 1970s, these discussions involved global health visionaries of their time, including Dame Nita Barrow, Jack Bryant,

Carl Taylor, and William Foege, all of whom were members of the CMC, and high-level officials at the World Health Organization (WHO), including Haldan Mahler, then Director–General, and Ken Newell, Director of Strengthening of Health Services at WHO [20,21]. One of the fruits of these discussions was the seminal WHO publication, *Health by the People* [22]. This book described a number of successful pioneering CBPHC projects around the world and laid the groundwork for the 1978 International Conference on Primary Health Care at Alma–Ata, Kazakhstan and the now renowned Declaration of Alma–Ata, which called for Health for All by the Year 2000 through primary health care [21,23].

Article V of the 1978 Declaration of Alma–Ata states the following [24]:

"Governments have a responsibility for the health of their people that can be fulfilled only by the provision of adequate health and social measures. A main social target of governments, international organizations and the whole world community in the coming decades should be the attainment by all peoples of the world by the year 2000 of a level of health that will permit them to lead a socially and economically productive life. Primary health care is the key to attaining this target as part of development in the spirit of social justice."

The broad concept of primary health care articulated in this Declaration was much more than the delivery of medical services at primary health care centers. Primary health care, as defined by the Declaration of Alma–Ata, involves providing preventive, promotive, curative, and rehabilitative health care services as close to the community as possible by members of a health team, including community health workers and traditional practitioners, and it broadened the concept even further by calling for primary health care to also address the primary causes of ill–health through inter–sectoral collaboration, community participation, and reduction of inequities.

Over the past three decades since the Declaration of Alma–Ata, major progress has been made in reducing child and maternal mortality throughout the world. The number of children dying before 5 years of age has declined from 18.9 million in 1960 [25] to 5.9 million in 2015 [26] despite the fact that the number of births each year has increased from 96 million in 1960 [25] to 139 million in 2015 [27]. The global under–5 mortality rate has declined from 148 per 1000 live births in 1970 [25] to 43 in 2015 [26]. Over the past 25 years, the global under–5 mortality rate globally has fallen by 53% [26], far less than the 67% required to reach the Millennium Development Goal for 2015. Reductions in maternal mortality have also been important but more gradual. The number of maternal deaths declined from 532 000 in 1990 to 303 000 in 2015 [28], and the global maternal mortality ratio fell by 44% during this period [28], far less than the 75% required to achieve the Millennium Development Goal.

Although evidence about the effectiveness of specific community–based interventions is generally well–documented, evidence about the total range of CBPHC interventions for MNCH, their effectiveness, how these interventions are actually delivered in practice (particularly in combination with other interventions), and the conditions that appear to be important for achieving success are less summarized. This is the heart of what our review is about.

Our review begins with the premises that (1) further strengthening CBPHC by expanding the population coverage of evidence–based interventions has the potential to accelerate progress in ending preventable child and maternal deaths, and (2) CBPHC has the potential for providing an entry point for establishing a more comprehensive primary health care system in resource–constrained settings that can enable health systems to more effectively improve population health and, at the same time, more effectively meet the needs and expectations of local people for medical care.

There is now, more than ever, a need for evaluation of what works and for "systematic sharing of good practices and greater sharing of new information" [29]. As an editorial in *The Lancet* [30] observed:

"Evaluation must now become the top priority in global health. Currently, it is only an afterthought. A massive scale–up in global health investments during the past decade has not been matched by an equal commitment to evaluation.... [Evaluation] will not only sustain interest in global health. It will improve quality of decision making, enhance efficiency, and build capacity for understanding why some programmes work and others do not. Evaluation matters. Evaluation is science."

This series provides an opportunity to summarize, review and analyze the evidence regarding the effectiveness of CBPHC in improving the health of mothers and their children, to draw conclusions regarding the findings from this review, and to suggest next steps in research, policy and program implementation.

Background of the review

In the early 1990s, Dr John Wyon (now deceased) and Dr Henry Perry organized panels at the annual meetings of the American Public Health Association (APHA) to highlight the contributions of CBPHC to improving the health of geographically–defined populations. As a result of support and encouragement from the International Health Section at APHA and from APHA staff, a Working Group on CBPHC within the International Health Section was established in 1997. For two decades now, the Working Group has been holding day–long annual workshops on themes related to CBPHC. One of these workshops led to the publication of a book on CBPHC [31]. As the evidence continued to mount regarding the effectiveness of CBPHC in improving health, the Working Group decided that a comprehensive review was needed.

Thus, beginning in 2005, the Working Group created a Task Force for the Review of the Evidence of CBPHC in Improving Child Health, with Henry Perry and Paul Freeman serving as Co–Chairs. What began as a small volunteer effort by Perry and Freeman and others has now, more than a decade later, involved over 150 people and not only APHA but also the World Health Organization, UNICEF, the World Bank, the US Agency for International Development, Future Generations (the NGO where Dr Perry was employed at the outset of the review), and most recently the Gates Foundation.

Following an initial small grant from the World Health Organization in 2006, an Expert Panel was created under the chairmanship of Dr Carl Taylor, then Professor Emeritus of International Health at the Johns Hopkins University (**Table 1**). This group participated in the initial design of the review and then later met face to face at UNICEF Headquarters in 2008 to discuss preliminary findings of the review. After Dr Taylor's death in 2010, the Panel reconvened under the leadership of Dr Robert Black, Professor of International Health at Johns Hopkins, and has participated in the final set of recommendations that constitute the final article in this series [32].

When the review began in 2006, the focus was exclusively on child health (that is, the health of children in their first 5 years of life). With support from USAID and the Gates Foundation between 2013 and 2016, it became possible to expand the scope of the review to maternal health. Thus, we have now renamed the overall effort a review of the effectiveness of CBPHC in improving MNCH.

Goals of the review

The goal of this review is to summarize the evidence regarding what can be achieved through community–based approaches to improve MNCH. The health of mothers, neonates and children as a measurable outcome is defined here for our purposes as the level of mortality, serious morbidity, nutritional status, or coverage of proven interventions for mothers, neonates and children in a geographically defined population. The review focuses on interventions and approaches that are carried out beyond the walls of health facilities that serve populations of mothers, neonates and children living in geographically defined areas.

Table 1. *Members of the Expert Panel for the Review of the Effectiveness of Community–Based Primary Health Care in Improving Maternal, Neonatal and Child Health*

Name	Organizational affiliation	Title	Location	Participated in formalization of guidelines for review 2006	Participated in face–to–face meeting of Panel in 2008	Participated in review of final findings (2016)
Raj Arole	Jamkhed Comprehensive Rural Health Project	Director (now deceased)	Jamkhed, India	X		
Shobha Arole	Jamkhed Comprehensive Rural Health Project	Director	Jamkhed, India			X
Rajiv Bahl	World Health Organization	Medical Officer, Child and Adolescent Health and Development Unit	Geneva, Switzerland	X		
Abhay Bang	Society for Education, Action and Research in Community Health (SEARCH)	Director	Gadchiroli, India	X	X	X
Al Bartlett	United States Agency for International Development	Formerly Senior Advisor for Child Survival, USAID; now retired	Washington, DC, USA	X		
Zulfiqar Bhutta	Centre for Global Child Health, Hospital for Sick Children, Toronto, Canada and Center of Excellence in Women and Child Health, the Aga Khan University, Karachi, Pakistan	Professor	Toronto, Canada and Karachi, Pakistan			X
Robert Black*	Bloomberg School of Public Health, Johns Hopkins University	Professor, Department of International Health	Baltimore, MD, USA	X	X	X
Mushtaque Chowdhury	BRAC	Formerly Dean of the James Grant School of Public Health; currently Deputy Director	Dhaka, Bangladesh			X

Table 1. *Continued*

Name	Organizational affiliation	Title	Location	Participated in formalization of guidelines for review 2006	Participated in face–to–face meeting of Panel in 2008	Participated in review of final findings (2016)
Anthony Costello	World Health Organization	Formerly Professor, International Perinatal Care Unit, Institute of Child Health, University College, London; currently Director, Department of Maternal, Newborn, Child and Adolescent Health	Geneva, Switzerland	X		
Dan Kaseje	Tropical Institute of Community Health and Development	Director	Kisumu, Kenya	X	X	X
Betty Kirkwood	London School of Hygiene and Tropical Medicine	Public Health Intervention Research Unit, Professor of Epidemiology and International Health	London, England	X		X
Rudolph Knippenberg	UNICEF	Senior Advisor for Health	New York, NY, USA	X	X	
Nazo Kureshy	United States Agency for International Development	Team Leader, Child Survival and Health Grants Program, Bureau for Global Health	Washington, DC, USA		X	X
Claudio Lanata	Instituto de Investigation Nutricional	Senior Researcher	Lima, Peru	X	X	X
Adetokunbo Lucas	Harvard University	Adjunct Professor of International Health	Ibidan, Nigeria	X	X	
James Phillips	Mailman School of Public Health, Columbia University	Professor	New York, NY, USA	X	X	X
Pang Ruyan	School of Public Health, Peking University	Visiting Professor and formerly National Coordinator for China, WHO Global Survey on Maternal and Perinatal Health	Beijing, China	X	X	
David Sanders	School of Public Health, University of Western Cape	Professor and Dean emeritus	Cape Town, South Africa	X	X	

Table 1. *Continued*

Name	Organizational affiliation	Title	Location	Participated in formalization of guidelines for review 2006	Participated in face-to-face meeting of Panel in 2008	Participated in review of final findings (2016)
Agnes Soucat	World Health Organization	Formerly Lead Economist, Human Development, Africa Region of the World Bank and currently Director of Health Systems, Governance and Financing of the World Health Organization	Geneva, Switzerland	X		
Carl Taylor†	Bloomberg School of Public Health, Johns Hopkins University	Professor Emeritus, Department of International Health (now deceased)	Baltimore, MD, USA	X	X	
Mary Taylor	Independent consultant	Formerly Senior Program Officer, Community Health Solutions, the Gates Foundation and currently Independent Senior Technical Expert	South Royalton, Vermont, USA	X	X	X
Cesar Victora	Federal University of Pelotas	Professor of Epidemiology	Pelotas, Brazil	X		X
Zonghan Zhu	Capital Institute of Pediatrics and China Advisory Center for Child Health, Beijing; Chinese Preventive Medicine Association	Professor, Capital Institute of Pediatrics and China Advisory Center for Child Health, Beijing, and Chairman of Child Health, Chinese Preventive Medicine Association	Beijing, China	X	X	X

*Chair of the Panel, 2010 to present.
†Chair of the Panel, 2006–2010.

The review consists of an analysis of documents describing research studies, field projects, and programs (collectively referred to in this series as projects) that have assessed the impact of CBPHC on MNCH. Altogether, the findings comprise a comprehensive overview of the global evidence in using CBPHC to improve MNCH. In addition, the review describes the strategies used to deliver community–based interventions and the role of the community and community health workers in implementing these interventions. In addition, the review seeks to understand the context of the projects – where they were implemented and by whom, where the funding came from, for how long, what size of population was served by the project, and what additional contextual factors might have influenced the project outcomes – as well as the methodological quality of the assessment.

The questions which the review seeks to answer are:

- How strong is the evidence that CBPHC can improve MNCH in geographically defined populations and sustain that improvement?
- What specific CBPHC activities improve MNCH?
- What conditions (including those within the local health system) facilitate the effectiveness of CBPHC and what community–based approaches appear to be most effective?
- What characteristics do effective CBPHC activities share?
- What program elements are correlated with improvements in child and maternal health?
- How strong is the evidence that partnerships between communities and health systems are required in order to improve child and maternal health?
- How strong is the evidence that CBPHC can promote equity?
- What general lessons can be drawn from the findings of this review?
- What additional research is needed?
- How can successful community–based approaches for improving MNCH be scaled up to regional and national levels within the context of serious financial and human resource constraints?
- What are the implications for local, national and global health policy, for program implementation, and for donors?

METHODS

The Task Force and the Expert Panel agreed on the following definition of CBPHC:

CBPHC is a process through which health programs and communities work together to improve health and control disease. CBPHC includes the promotion of key behaviors at the household level as well as the provision of health care and health services outside of health facilities at the community level. CBPHC can (and of course should) connect to existing health services, health programs, and health care provided at static facilities (including health centers and hospitals) and be closely integrated with them.

CBPHC involves improving the health of a geographically defined population through outreach outside of health facilities. CBPHC does not include health care provided at a health facility unless there is community involvement and associated services beyond the facility.

CBPHC also includes multi–sectoral approaches to health improvement beyond the provision of health services per se, including programs that seek to improve (directly or indirectly) education, income, nutrition, living standards, and empowerment.

CBPHC programs may or may not collaborate with governmental or private health care programs; they may be comprehensive in scope, highly selective, or somewhere in between; and they may or may not be part of a program which includes the provision of services at health facilities.

CBPHC includes the following three different types of interventions:
- Health communication with individuals, families and communities;
- Social mobilization and community involvement for planning, delivering, evaluating and using health services; and
- Provision of health care in the community, including preventive services (eg, immunizations) or curative services (eg, community–based treatment of pneumonia).

Types of assessments of maternal, neonatal and child health interventions qualifying for review

The Task Force sought documents that described community–based programs, projects and research studies that carried out assessments of changes in MNCH indicators in such a way that any changes observed could reasonably be attributed to CBPHC program interventions. At least one of the following outcome indicators was required to be present in order for the assessment to be included in the review.

Maternal health
- Change in the population coverage of one or more evidence–based interventions (utilization of antenatal care, delivery by a trained attendant, delivery in a health facility, clean delivery, and postpartum care)
- Change in nutritional status
- Change in the incidence or in the outcome of serious, life–threatening morbidity (such as pre–eclampsia, eclampsia, sepsis, hemorrhage); or,
- Change in mortality.

Neonatal and child health

- Change in the population coverage of one or more evidence–based interventions (clean delivery; appropriate care during the neonatal period; appropriate infant and young child feeding, including appropriate breastfeeding; immunizations; vitamin A supplementation; appropriate prevention of malaria with insecticide–treated bed nets and intermittent preventive therapy; appropriate hand washing; appropriate treatment of drinking water, appropriate sanitation; appropriate treatment of pneumonia, diarrhea and malaria;
- Change in nutritional status (as measured by anthropometry, anemia, or assessment of micro–nutrient deficiency);
- Change in the incidence or in the outcome of serious but non–life–threatening morbidity (such as trachoma, which can result in blindness);
- Change in the incidence or in the outcome of serious, life–threatening morbidity (such as pneumonia, diarrhea, malaria, and low–birth weight); or,
- Change in mortality (perinatal, neonatal, infant, 1–4–year, and under–5 mortality);

In addition, the review included an analysis of available documentation concerning the degree to which improvements in child health obtained by CBPHC approaches were equitable.

Document retrieval

The principal inclusion criteria for the literature review were: (1) a report describing the CBPHC program for a defined geographic population and (2) a description of the findings of an assessment of the project's effect on maternal, neonatal or child health as defined above. The focus was on the effectiveness of program interventions on the health of all mothers and/or children in a geographically defined area, although in some cases (eg, in studies of maternal–to–child HIV transmission), the focus was on a subset of mothers and their children in a geographically defined area.

Key terms for "maternal health," "child health," "community health," and "developing countries" and related terms were identified to create a search query (see Tables S1 and S2 in **Online Supplementary Document**). The United States National Library of Medicine's PubMed database was searched periodically up until 31 December 2015 using these two queries, yielding 7890 articles on maternal health and 4276 articles on neonatal or child health (**Figure 1**). The articles were screened separately by two members of the study team. Assessments of the effectiveness of CBPHC in which the outcomes were improvements in neurological, emotional or psychological development of children were not included unless the reports also included one or more of the other neonatal or child health outcome measures mentioned above.

In addition to the PubMed search, broadcasts were sent out on widely used global health listservs, including those of the Global Health Council, the American Public Health Association, the Collaboration and Resources Group for Child Health (the CORE Group), the World Federation of Public Health Associations, and the Association of Schools of Public Health asking for information about documents, reports, and published articles which might qualify for the review. Finally, the Task Force contacted knowledgeable persons in the field for their suggestions for documents to be included, including members of the Expert Panel. Documents not published in peer–reviewed scientific journals were included if they met the criteria for review, if they provided an adequate description of the intervention, and if they had a satisfactory form of evaluation. A total of 152 assessments met the criteria for the maternal health review and 548 for the neonatal/child health review (**Figure 1**).

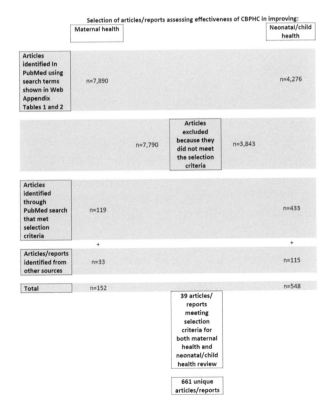

Figure 1. *Selection process of assessments of the effectiveness of community-based primary health care (CBPHC).*

Table S3 in **Online Supplementary Document** contains a bibliography with the references associated with these 700 assessments. The bibliography also indicates which references were in the maternal health review, in the child health review (and which of these were included in the analyses for neonatal health and child health), and the equity review. There are a number of cases in which a single assessment in our database is derived from more than one document. All of these references are included in the bibliography. Thus, when in **Figure 1** above we refer to the number of articles/reports, there are a small number of cases in which we have combined the various articles/ reports associated with a single assessment and counted this as only one assessment.

Of the 33 maternal health assessments and the 115 neonatal/child health assessments included in the review that were not identified through PubMed, most (16 and 80, respectively) were project evaluations of child survival projects funded by the USAID Child Survival and Health Grants Program and implemented by US–based non–governmental organizations. These are listed separately in Table S4 in **Online Supplementary Document.** Other assessments that were not identified through PubMed were evaluations from other sources, books, or book chapters.

The document review process

Two data extraction forms were prepared through an iterative process. The extraction form to be used for child health assessments and the form for maternal health assessments were identical except for the interventions carried out. These forms are contained in Appendices S5 and S6 in **Online Supplementary Document**. Both forms were developed with the purpose of extracting all possible information available regarding how the interventions were implemented at the community level and what the role of the community was in implementation.

Two independent reviewers each completed a Data Extraction Form for each assessment that qualified for the review. A third reviewer provided quality control and resolved any difference observed in the two reviews, and the final summative review was transferred to an EPI INFO database (version 3.5.4) (Epi Info, US Centers for Disease Control and Prevention, Atlanta, Georgia, USA). The names of the reviewers, many of whom worked on a volunteer basis, are shown in the acknowledgment section; their names and professional titles are contained in Table S7 in **Online Supplementary Document**.

Comment on terminology used

The assessments included in our review were carried out for field studies, projects, and programs that employed one or more CBPHC interventions for improving maternal, neonatal and/or child health. This is a heterogeneous group of assessments in the sense that they range from (1) research reports describing the efficacy of single interventions over a short period of time in a highly supervised and well–supported field setting to (2) assessments of programs which provided a comprehensive array of health and development programs over a long period of time in more typical field setting. When referring to this group of community–level activities as a whole, they should properly be referred to as "research studies/field projects/programs" but for practicality's sake we will refer to them throughout this series simply as "projects," and the evaluations of their effectiveness as "assessments."

Database description

An electronic database describing 700 assessments of the effectiveness of CB-PHC in improving MNCH was queried using EPI INFO version 3.5.4 and STA-TA version 14 (StatCorp LLC, College Station, Texas, USA). For the purpose of this review, the 39 assessments with both maternal and child health outcomes have been counted as separate assessments in our analysis. Overall, 78.8% of assessments are scientific articles published in peer–reviewed journals, 4.0% are some other type of publication (mostly books or reports not available on the internet), and 12.7% are either from the gray literature (available on the internet) or unpublished project evaluations.

Over three–fourths (78.4%) of the assessments included in our review were carried out in rural settings at least in part, while 16.9% and 11.1% were carried out exclusively in an urban or peri–urban setting, respectively.

Among the 700 assessments in our data set, a small proportion contained data from more than one country. Thus, altogether, 786 country–specific assessments were identified. India, Bangladesh, and Nepal had the largest number of assessments (86, 77, and 47, respectively). 49.0% of the country–specific assessments came from Africa WHO Region, 28.5% from the South–East Asia Region, and 9.7% from the Americas (**Table 2** and Table S8 in **Online Supplementary Document**). 8.6% of reports assessed interventions in a single community, 38.1% in a set of communities not encompassing an entire health district (or sub–province), 37.5% at the district (or sub–province) level, 7.5% at the provincial/state level, 3.7% at a national level, and 3.2% at a multinational level.

Table 2. *Number of assessments of the effectiveness of community–based primary health care in improving maternal, neonatal and child health by region and the countries with the greatest number of assessments*

WHO REGION	NUMBER	% (N = 786)*	COUNTRY	NUMBER	% (N = 786)*
Africa	385	49.0%	India	86	10.9
South–East Asia	224	28.5%	Bangladesh	77	9.8
Americas	76	9.7%	Nepal	47	6.0
Eastern Mediterranean	61	7.8%	Ghana	36	4.6
Western Pacific	37	4.7%	Pakistan	35	4.5
Europe	4	0.5%	Uganda	34	4.3
Total	786*	100.0%	Tanzania	30	3.8
			Ethiopia	28	3.6
			Kenya	27	3.4
			Malawi	19	2.4

*The total number of countries listed here exceeds the number of assessments because some assessments were conducted in multiple countries.

The implementing and facilitating organizations for these projects were primarily private entities (NGOs, universities and research organizations), often working with governments at the national, provincial, or local level (**Table 3**). While communities were — by definition — involved in all of these projects, in only 4.3% of assessments were local communities the only identified implementers. Those who actually implemented projects at the local level were community health workers (CHWs), local community members, research workers, and government health staff.

Half (49.3%) of the assessments are of projects serving 5000 or fewer women and children. 18.2% of the assessments are based on data derived from projects reaching more than 25 000 women and children. 61.9% of the projects had begun since 2000. Almost half (46.3%) of projects were less than 2 years in duration and almost two–thirds (62.9%) were implemented for less than 3 years. Among the neonatal and child health assessments, 51.6% were of only one intervention, and 87.4% were of four or fewer interventions. On the other hand, among the maternal health assessments three–quarters (75.7%) included five or more interventions.

Our review includes 16 assessments of projects that were completed before 1980. The earliest report describes the health impact of an integrated primary health care project in South Africa led by Sidney Kark in the 1940s and published in 1952 [33]. The next earliest report concerns the effectiveness of tetanus toxoid immunization in Columbia, South America, published in 1966 [34].

Table 3. *Implementers of projects for improving MNCH*

	NUMBER	% (N = 700)
Facilitating and/or stakeholder organization:		
State or national government	424	60.6
International NGO	281	40.1
Private organization/university/research organization	254	36.3
Local government	243	34.7
Local NGO	125	17.9
National NGO	85	12.1
Faith–based organization	27	3.9
Implementers at the community level:		
Community health workers (either paid or volunteer)	519	74.1
Research workers only for the project	238	34.0
Ministry of health worker or other government–paid health workers/ professionals	304	43.4
Local community members (not trained as a CHW)	200	28.6
Expatriates	33	4.7

*Percentages add up to more than 100% because projects often utilized more than one Implementer.

Number of assessments completed over time

There has been a rapid growth in the number of assessments published between 1980 and 2015, but particularly in the period 2001–2011, the decade following the establishment of the Millennium Development Goals (MDGs) (**Figure 2**). The surge in publications is present both for maternal and for child/neonatal health studies (data not shown). In the five years from 2011 until the

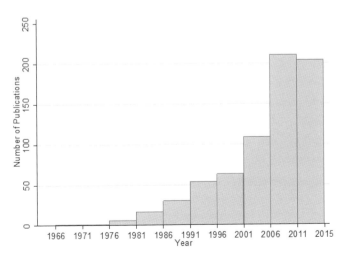

Figure 2. *Number of assessments in data set by year of publication (in 5-year intervals).*

end of 2015 when the assessment retrieval ended, there was a slight decline in the number of publications.

Types of outcomes assessed

We identified a total of 239 outcomes measured in the 700 assessments included in the review: 56 maternal outcomes and 183 neonatal/child outcomes (see Tables S7 and S8 in **Online Supplementary Document**). Common maternal health outcomes were changes in: mortality, receipt of antenatal care, attendance at delivery by a skilled provider, facility delivery, care for obstetric emergencies, receipt of nutritional supplements, receipt of tetanus toxoid vaccination, receipt of post–partum family planning, knowledge of safe birth practices, and screening for HIV and other sexually transmitted infections during pregnancy. Common neonatal and child health outcomes were: changes in mortality, serious morbidity, nutritional status, population coverage of healthy behaviors, and changes in the appropriate utilization of health services. In addition, some assessments contained outcome measures that did not qualify for the review but were included with other indicators that did qualify for the review. These include progress in psychomotor development, changes in health–related knowledge among parents and caretakers, quality of community case management of acute childhood illness provided by CHWs, and measures of improvements in health system capacity.

Types of research methodologies used to assess effectiveness

In the majority (61.0%) of the assessments, a control or comparison group was present. In almost three–fourths (72.5%), pre– and post–intervention data were collected. In 44.6% of the assessments, both data from a comparison group as well as pre– and post–intervention data were present. Randomized controlled assessment designs were present in 33.7% of the assessments. 27.4% of the assessments were uncontrolled before–after assessment designs. Reviewers considered the methodology to be adequate in 89.8% of the assessments, and they considered the assessment quality to be good, high, or exceptional for 88.4% of the assessments.

Source of financial support for assessments

The United States Agency for International Development (USAID) was far and away the largest source of financial support for the assessments included in our review, contributing to the financial support of one–third (33.4%) of the assessments included in the review. UNICEF supported the next largest number of assessments (15.8%), followed by the World Health Organization (14.2%), the Gates Foundation (10.7%), other UN agencies (7.7%), and the World Bank (6.2%) (**Table 4**). There were numerous other donors that funded a smaller number of assessments. In most (but not all) cases, the donor funded the project as well as the assessment.

Table 4. *Leading sources of financial support for projects whose assessments were included in the database*

Donor	Number of projects/assessments supported	% (n = 700)*
US Agency for International Development	233	33.3
UNICEF	110	15.7
World Health Organization (including the Pan American Health Organization)	99	14.1
The Bill and Melinda Gates Foundation	75	10.7
Other UN agency (eg, UNDP, UNFPA, UNHCR, WFP)	54	7.7
World Bank	43	6.1
Department for International Development (UK)	28	4.0
Canadian International Development Agency (CIDA)	23	3.3
Wellcome Trust	18	2.6

*Multiple funders may have supported a single project/assessment.

Availability of the database for further analyses and potential further development of the database

We are not aware of any other similar database in existence. It serves as the basis for the subsequent articles in this series [32,35–40]. However, there is an opportunity for more analyses of the database than is reported in this series. Any of the project assessments included in this review are available to be shared with anyone who is interested (contact Henry Perry at hperry2@jhu.edu).

The potential exists for maintaining this as a dynamic database that is regularly updated and publicly available. And, the potential also exists for expanding this database beyond MNCH to include community–based approaches to other global health priorities such as HIV, tuberculosis, malaria, and chronic diseases.

Limitations of the review

Our review is a comprehensive one, but we make no claim that it is a complete or systematic review. Resources and time constraints prevented screening other electronic databases beyond PubMed for reports that met the inclusion criteria. In addition, the USAID Child Survival and Health Grants program has an archive of more than 400 unpublished child survival project evaluations that meet the criteria for inclusion and are publicly available, but resource and time constraints were such that only one–fifth (80) of these could be included in our review. Since the data analysis and write up portion of this study began, we have identified several additional articles that would have qualified for the review. However, none of these would have changed the overall findings of our review.

This review is limited to documents that describe the impact of project interventions. As is well–known, program failures and serious challenges encountered in program implementation are rarely described in open–access documents or in the scientific literature. This means that a serious publication bias is present and should be recognized. Nonetheless, the inability to document these experiences does not detract from the value of the numerous assessments that have been included in our review that demonstrate effectiveness of CBPHC in improving MNCH.

The degree to which the assessments included in our review represent efficacy assessments as compared to effectiveness assessments is an important issue which we are not able to adequately explore. Efficacy assessments, of course, are carried out for projects that have been implemented under ideal circumstances, when field staff members have optimal training, supervision, resources, and logistical support, and when optimal community engagement has been established. These are conditions that often do not occur in routine settings. Effectiveness assessments, in contrast to efficacy assessments, are carried out under "real world" conditions. Our data extraction form did not collect information on this issue and, in fact, it is often difficult to determine exactly where a project might lie on a continuum between these end points. But it is the case that very few of the assessments in our database were of projects that were implemented without some type of international donor support or technical assistance. Thus, the database is not representative of the effectiveness of current day–to–day practice of CBPHC but rather of what has been achieved in special circumstances in which documentation of effectiveness was undertaken and in which presumably extra efforts had been made to assure the highest quality of implementation possible under the circumstances.

The degree to which these projects improved MNCH depended on many factors: the type(s) and number of interventions implemented, the quality of implementation, and myriad contextual factors. And, of course, the type of outcome indicator(s) employed is important as well. Given the heterogeneity of (1) the types of interventions implemented, (2) the manner in which they were implemented, and (3) the outcome measures used to assess outcomes, it is difficult to make definitive statements about the strength of the evidence, about the magnitude of effect for any specific intervention, or about the effectiveness of one specific approach to implementation compared to another. Rather, the aim of our study is to review the broad scope of evidence related to the effectiveness of CBPHC in improving MNCH and to draw conclusions about the overall effectiveness of CBPHC, the most common strategies used in implementation, and the potential for further strengthening of CBPHC to improve MNCH globally.

It is well–known that the use of family planning, birth spacing, and the reduction of unmet need for family planning all have favorable benefits for MNCH. Furthermore, the evidence on the effectiveness of CBPHC in increasing the coverage of family planning services is extensive. Thus, inclusion of this literature would have made our review more complete, but time and resources were not sufficient to carry this out.

Finally, our review has not included the effectiveness of CBPHC in reducing miscarriages and stillbirths. This topic is an important one but time and resources were not sufficient to carry this out either.

Subsequent articles in this series

Seven subsequent articles are being published in this series that answer the questions posed by the review. These include: (i) an analysis of the effectiveness of CBPHC in improving maternal health [35], (ii) an analysis of the effectiveness of CBPHC in improving neonatal health [36], (iii) an analysis of the effectiveness of CBPHC in improving child health [37], (iv) an analysis of the effectiveness of CBPHC in promoting equitable improvements in child health [40], (v) the strategies employed by effective CBPHC programs for achieving improvements in MNCH [38], (vi) an analysis of the common characteristics of integrated projects with long–term evidence of effectiveness in improving MNCH [39], and (vii) summary and recommendations of the Expert Panel [32].

CONCLUSIONS

An extensive database of the evidence regarding the effectiveness of CBPHC in improving MNCH has been assembled. Special attention has been given to how projects were implemented at the community level. The articles that follow in this series describe the findings of analyses of this database along with conclusions and recommendations of an Expert Panel. The aim of this series is to contribute to the formulation of policies and programs that will be useful for ending preventable maternal, neonatal and child deaths and for achieving universal access to care for women and their children by the year 2030 by strengthening CBPHC.

Acknowledgments: We are grateful to the following organizations that provided small grants to cover the expenses of this review: UNICEF, the World Bank, the Department of Child and Adolescent Health and Development of the World Health Organization, the CORE Group (Collaboration and Resources for Child Health)/USAID, Future Generations, and the Gates Foundation. We are also grateful to the American Public Health Association and particularly its International Health Section staff, which administered some of these funds. We thank Future Generations for providing office space, administrative support, and salary support to Dr Perry during the initial phase of the review. The World Bank made it possible for one of its consultants, Dr Bahie Rassekh, to participate as a member of the Study Team. We thank the following people for serving as reviewers of assessments: Binita Adhikari, Asma Aftab, Azal Ahmadi, Iain Aitken, Laura Altobelli, Chidinma Anakwenze, Ramin Asgary, Ann Ashworth Hill, Gretchen Berggren, Warren Berggren, Claire Boswell, Lisa Bowen, Amberle Brown, Jack Bryant, Juraci Cesar, Elizabeth Chan, Stephanie Chang, Elizabeth Cheatham, Ketan Chitnis, Len Christie, Deanna Crouse, Christine Davachi, Jean Richard Dortonne, Duane Dowell, Ashkan Emami, Sheila Enoh, Qi Fan, Meredith Fort, Paul Freeman, Asha George, Juliana Grant, Stacy Grau, Sundeep Gupta, Nancy Habarta, Nowreen Haq, Runa Haq, Paymon Hashemi, Ann Hershberger, Zelee Hill, Sandy Hoar, Asim Jani, Dennis Kim, Woon Cho Kim, Ajoy Kumar, Stacy Laswell, Ramiro Llanque, Amanda Long, Ron Mataya, Colin McCord, Meredith McMorrow, Henri Menager, Raul Mendoza–Sassi, William Menson, Pierre–Marie Metangmo, Gita Mirchandani, Mary Morgan, Lenna Neat, Oluwatosin Ogundalu, Pat Paredes, Vikash Parekh, Carlo Passeri, Zohra Patel, Erika Perez, Henry Perry, Laura Podewils, Jon Poehlman, Ramaswamy Premkumar, Braveen Ragunanthan, Bahie Mary Rassekh, James Ricca, Jeeva Rima, Jon Rohde, Evan Russell, Emma Sacks, Kwame Sakyi, Juan Sanchez, Nirali Shah, Manjunath Shankar, Mona Sharan, Donna Sillan, Stephen Stake, Laura Steinhardt, Parminder Suchdev, Mariame Sylla, Meghan Tamarro, Henry Taylor, Muyiwa Tegbe, Angeline Ti, Charles Teller, Yetsa Tuakli, Jess Wilhelm, Olga Wollinka, and Jean Yuan. Most of them helped as unpaid volunteers. Further information about them is contained in Table S5 of the online supplementary document. Binita Adhikari, Omar Balsara, David Exe, Pam Flynn, Jennifer Hutain, Mary Carol Jennings, Mirlene Perry, Elizabeth Randolph, Meike Schleiff provided assistance with assembling the database and inputting it into an electronic format. Claire Twose provided expert technical assistance for the computerized literature search. We thank them all. The organizations that provided financial support had no role in the execution of the review.

Funding: The following organizations provided funds that were used to conduct the work described in this article: The World Health Organization, UNICEF, the World Bank, the United States Agency for International Development, and the Gates Foundation. The organizations that provided financial support had no role in the execution of the review.

Authorship declaration: HP wrote the first draft. HP, PF, BR, and SG guided this project from the beginning to the end and participated in all decisions related to the overall review. JS performed the analysis of the quantitative data included in our report. All of the authors participated in the revision of earlier drafts and approved the final draft.

Conflict of interest: All authors have completed the Unified Competing Interest Form at www.icmje.org/coi_disclosure.pdf (available upon request from the corresponding author), and declare no conflict of interest.

References

1 Jones G, Steketee RW, Black RE, Bhutta ZA, Morris SS. How many child deaths can we prevent this year? Lancet. 2003;362:65-71. Medline:12853204 doi:10.1016/S0140-6736(03)13811-1

2 Hill Z, Kirkwood B, Edmond K. Family and community practices that promote child survival, growth and development: a review of the evidence. Geneva: World Health Organization; 2004.

3 Lassi ZS, Kumar R, Bhutta ZA. Community-based care to improve maternal, newborn, and child health. 2016. In: Disease Control Priorities: Reproductive, Maternal, Newborn, and Child Health, Third Edition. Washington, DC: World Bank. Available: https://openknowledge.worldbank.org/bitstream/handle/10986/23833/9781464803482.pdf?sequence=3&isAllowed=y26 February 2017. Accessed: 27 February 2017.

4 Bhutta ZA, Black RE. Global maternal, newborn, and child health–so near and yet so far. N Engl J Med. 2013;369:2226-35. Medline:24304052 doi:10.1056/NEJMra1111853

5 Black RE, Levin C, Walker N, Chou D, Liu L, Temmerman M, et al. Reproductive, maternal, newborn, and child health: key messages from Disease Control Priorities 3rd Edition. Lancet. 2016;388:2811-24.

6 Victora CG, Requejo JH, Barros AJ, Berman P, Bhutta Z, Boerma T, et al. Countdown to 2015: a decade of tracking progress for maternal, newborn, and child survival. Lancet. 2016;387:2049-59. Medline:26477328 doi:10.1016/S0140-6736(15)00519-X

7 Bhutta ZA, Darmstadt GL, Hasan BS, Haws RA. Community-based interventions for improving perinatal and neonatal health outcomes in developing countries: a review of the evidence. Pediatrics. 2005;115(2 Suppl):519-617. Medline:15866863 doi:10.1542/peds.2004-1441

8 Freeman P, Perry HB, Gupta SK, Rassekh B. Accelerating progress in achieving the millennium development goal for children through community-based approaches. Glob Public Health. Glob Public Health. 2012;7:400-19. Medline:19890758 doi:10.1080/17441690903330305

9 Bhutta ZA, Lassi ZS, Pariyo G, Huicho L. Global experience of Community Health Workers for delivery of health related Millennium Development Goals: a systematic review, country case studies, and recommendation for integration into national health systems. Geneva: World Health Organization and the Global Health Workforce Alliance; 2010. Available: http://www.who.int/workforcealliance/knowledge/publications/alliance/Global_CHW_web.pdf. Accessed: 26 February 2017.

10 Gogia S, Sachdev HS. Home visits by community health workers to prevent neonatal deaths in developing countries: a systematic review. Bull World Health Organ. 2010;88:658-66B. Medline:20865070 doi:10.2471/BLT.09.069369

11 Kidney E, Winter HR, Khan KS, Gulmezoglu AM, Meads CA, Deeks JJ, et al. Systematic review of effect of community-level interventions to reduce maternal mortality. BMC Pregnancy Childbirth. 2009;9:2. Medline:19154588 doi:10.1186/1471-2393-9-2

12 Lassi ZS, Haider BA, Bhutta ZA. Community-based intervention packages for reducing maternal and neonatal morbidity and mortality and improving neonatal outcomes. Cochrane Database Syst Rev. 2010;11:CD007754. Medline:21069697

13 Lewin S, Munabi-Babigumira S, Glenton C, Daniels K, Bosch-Capblanch X, van Wyk BE, et al. Lay health workers in primary and community health care for maternal and child health and the management of infectious diseases. Cochrane Database Syst Rev. 2010;3:CD004015. Medline:20238326

14 Salam RA, Haroon S, Ahmed HH, Das JK, Bhutta ZA. Impact of community-based interventions on HIV knowledge, attitudes, and transmission. Infect Dis Poverty. 2014;3:26. Medline:25126420 doi:10.1186/2049-9957-3-26

15 Sazawal S, Black RE. Effect of pneumonia case management on mortality in neonates, infants, and preschool children: a meta-analysis of community-based trials. Lancet Infect Dis. 2003;3:547-56. Medline:12954560 doi:10.1016/S1473-3099(03)00737-0

16 Schiffman J, Darmstadt GL, Agarwal S, Baqui AH. Community-based intervention packages for improving perinatal health in developing countries: a review of the evidence. Semin Perinatol. 2010;34:462-76. Medline:21094420 doi:10.1053/j.semperi.2010.09.008

17 Miller S, Abalos E, Chamillard M, Ciapponi A, Colaci D, Comande D, et al. Beyond too little, too late and too much, too soon: a pathway towards evidence-based, respectful maternity care worldwide. Lancet. 2016;388:2176-92. Medline:27642019 doi:10.1016/S0140-6736(16)31472-6

18 Chan M. Return to Alma-Ata. Lancet. 2008;372:865-6. Medline:18790292 doi:10.1016/S0140-6736(08)61372-0

19 Arole M, Kasaje D, Taylor C. The Christian Medical Commission's Role in the Worldwide Primary Health Care Movement. In: Taylor C, Desai A, Knutsson K, O'Dea-Knutsson P, Taylor-Ide D, editors. Partnerships for Social Development: A Casebook. Franklin, WV, USA: Future Generations; 1995.

20 Litsios S. The long and difficult road to Alma-Ata: a personal reflection. Int J Health Serv. 2002;32:709-32. Medline:12456122 doi:10.2190/RP8C-L5UB-4RAF-NRH2

21 Litsios S. The Christian Medical Commission and the development of the World Health Organization's primary health care approach. Am J Public Health. 2004;94:1884-93. Medline:15514223 doi:10.2105/AJPH.94.11.1884

22 Newell KW, editor. Health by the People. Geneva, Switzerland: World Health Organization; 1975.

23 WHO. UNICEF. Declaration of Alma-Ata. International Conference on Primary Health Care, Alma-Ata, USSR, 6-12 September 1978 Geneva, Switzerland: World Health Organization; 1978. Available: http://www.who.int/publications/almaata_declaration_en.pdf?ua=1. Accessed: 27 February 2017.

24 WHO. UNICEF (editors). International Conference on Primary Health Care, Alma Ata. 1978; USSR: World Health Organization, Geneva.

25 Ahmad OB, Lopez AD, Inoue M. The decline in child mortality: a reappraisal. Bull World Health Organ. 2000;78:1175-91. Medline:11100613

26 You D, Hug L, Ejdemyr S, Idele P, Hogan D, Mathers C, et al. Global, regional, and national levels and trends in under-5 mortality between 1990 and 2015, with scenario-based projections to 2030: a systematic analysis by the UN Inter-agency Group for Child Mortality Estimation. Lancet. 2015;386:2275-86. Medline:26361942 doi:10.1016/S0140-6736(15)00120-8

27 UNICEF. The State of the World's Children 2015: Reimagine the Future. Innovation for Every Child. New York: UNICEF; 2014. Available: http://sowc2015.unicef.org/. Accessed: 27 February 2017.

28 WHO, World Bank, UNICEF, UNFPA. Trends in Maternal Mortality: 1990 to 2015. 2015. World Health Organization. Available: http://apps.who.int/iris/bitstream/10665/194254/1/9789241565141_eng.pdf?ua=1. Accessed: 7 October 2016.

29 UNICEF. Tracking Progress in Maternal, Newborn and Child Survival. The 2008 Report New York: Geneva; 2008. Available: http://www.who.int/pmnch/Countdownto-2015FINALREPORT-apr7.pdf. Accessed: 27 February 2017.

30 Evaluation: the top priority for global health. Lancet. 2010;375:526. Medline:20079530 doi:10.1016/S0140-6736(10)60056-6

31 Rohde JE, Wyon J, editors. Community-Based Health Care: Lessons from Bangladesh to Boston. Boston, MA: Management Sciences for Health (in collaboration with the Harvard School of Public Health); 2002.

32 Black R. Taylor. C, Expert Panel. Comprehensive review of the evidence regarding the effectiveness of community-based primary health care in improving maternal, neonatal and child health: 8. conclusions and recommendations of an Expert Panel. J Glob Health. 2017;7:010908.

33 Kark SL, Cassel J. The Pholela Health Centre; a progress report. S Afr Med J. 1952;26:101-4. Medline:14913265

34 Newell KW, Duenas Lehmann A, LeBlanc DR, Garces Osorio N. The use of toxoid for the prevention of tetanus neonatorum. Final report of a double-blind controlled field trial. Bull World Health Organ. 1966;35:863-71. Medline:5338377

35 Jennings M, Pradhan S, Schleiff M, Sacks E, Freeman P, Gupta S, et al. Comprehensive review of the evidence regarding the effectiveness of community-based primary health care in improving maternal, neonatal and child health: 2. maternal health findings. J Glob Health. 2017;7:010902.

36 Sacks E, Freeman P, Sakyi K, Jennings M, Rassekh B, Gupta S, et al. Comprehensive review of the evidence regarding the effectiveness of community-based primary health care in improving maternal, neonatal and child health: 3. neonatal health findings. J Glob Health. 2017;7:010903.

37 Freeman P, Schleiff M, Sacks E, Rassekh B, Gupta S, Perry H. Comprehensive review of the evidence regarding the effectiveness of community-based primary health care in improving maternal, neonatal and child health: 4. child health findings. J Glob Health. 2017;7:010904.

38 Perry H, Rassekh B, Gupta S, Freeman P. Comprehensive review of the evidence regarding the effectiveness of community-based primary health care in improving maternal, neonatal and child health: 6. strategies used by effective projects. J Glob Health. 2017;7:010906.

39 Perry H, Rassekh B, Gupta S, Freeman P. Comprehensive review of the evidence regarding the effectiveness of community-based primary health care in improving maternal, neonatal and child health: 7. Programs with evidence of long-term impact on mortality in children younger than five years of age. J Glob Health. 2017;7:010907.

40 Schleiff M, Kumapley R, Freeman P, Gupta S, Rassekh B, Perry H. Comprehensive review of the evidence regarding the effectiveness of community-based primary health care in improving maternal, neonatal and child health: 5. equity effects. J Glob Health. 2017;7:010905.

Acknowledgement: originally published as: Henry B Perry, Bahie M Rassekh, Sundeep Gupta, Jess Wilhelm, Paul A Freeman:Comprehensive review of the evidence regarding the effectiveness of Community–Based Primary Health Care in improving maternal, neonatal and child health: 1. rationale, methods and database description. Reprinted with permission from Edinburgh University Global Health Society under Creative Commons Attribution Licence (Journal of Global Health 2017; 010901).

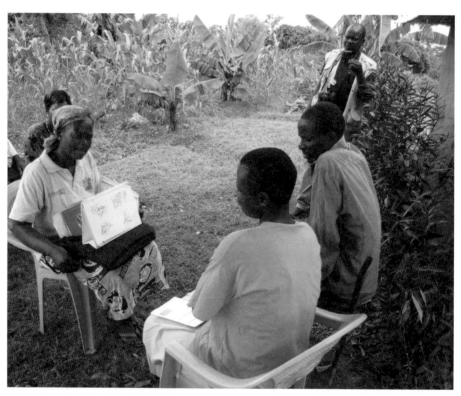

A volunteer community health worker visiting a mother and her husband
at their home in rural western Kenya
Photocredit: Henry Perry (used with permission).

A comprehensive review of the evidence regarding the effectiveness of community–based primary health care in improving maternal, neonatal and child health: 2. maternal health findings

Mary Carol Jennings[1], Subarna Pradhan[2], Meike Schleiff[1], Emma Sacks[1], Paul A Freeman[3,4], Sundeep Gupta[5], Bahie M Rassekh[6], Henry B Perry[1]

[1] Department of International Health, Johns Hopkins Bloomberg School of Public Health, Baltimore, MD, USA
[2] Institute for Global Health, Duke University, Durham, North Carolina, USA
[3] Independent Consultant, Seattle, Washington, USA
[4] Department of Global Health, University of Washington, Seattle, Washington, USA
[5] Medical Epidemiologist, Lusaka, Zambia
[6] The World Bank, Washington, District of Columbia, USA

Background We summarize the findings of assessments of projects, programs, and research studies (collectively referred to as projects) included in a larger review of the effectiveness of community–based primary health care (CBPHC) in improving maternal, neonatal and child health (MNCH). Findings on neonatal and child health are reported elsewhere in this series.

Methods We searched PUBMED and other databases through December 2015, and included assessments that underwent data extraction. Data were analyzed to identify themes in interventions implemented, health outcomes, and strategies used in implementation.

Results 152 assessments met inclusion criteria. The majority of assessments were set in rural communities. 72% of assessments included 1–10 specific interventions aimed at improving maternal health. A total of 1298 discrete interventions were assessed. Outcome measures were grouped into five main categories: maternal mortality (19% of assessments); maternal morbidity (21%); antenatal care attendance (50%); attended delivery (66%) and facility delivery (69%), with many assessments reporting results on multiple indicators. 15 assessment reported maternal mortality as a primary outcome, and of the seven that performed statistical testing, six reported significant decreases. Seven assessments measured changes in maternal morbidity: postpartum hemorrhage, malaria or eclampsia. Of those, six reported significant decreases and one did not find a significant effect. Assessments of community–based interventions on antenatal care attendance, attended delivery and facility–based deliveries all showed a positive impact. The community–based strategies used to achieve these results often involved community collaboration, home visits, formation of participatory women's groups, and provision of services by outreach teams from peripheral health facilities.

Conclusions This comprehensive and systematic review provides evidence of the effectiveness of CBPHC in improving key indicators of maternal morbidity and mortality. Most projects combined community– and facility–based approaches, emphasizing potential added benefits from such holistic approaches. Community–based interventions will be an important component of a comprehensive approach to accelerate improvements in maternal health and to end preventable maternal deaths by 2030.

Traditionally, maternal health programs in low–income settings have focused on improving the access to and quality of clinical services provided in health facilities. However, increasing facility delivery alone is likely insufficient for further substantial reductions in maternal mortality and morbidity [1,2]. The contribution that community–based primary health care (CBPHC) can make to improving maternal health has received much less attention. Although ready access to and appropriate utilization of primary health care centers and referral hospitals is essential to manage pregnancy complications [3,4], an increasing number of community–based interventions have been designed in an effort to accelerate improvements in maternal health.

Although improving maternal health by increasing the access to and the quality of maternal health care services has been acknowledged as a global health priority, recent progress in improving maternal health in low–income countries has been discouragingly slow, particularly in sub–Saharan Africa and parts of South Asia [5]. The Millennium Development Goal 5 (reducing maternal mortality by 75% between 1990 and 2015) was not met: only a 44% decline has been achieved globally – representing a decline from 385 to 216 maternal deaths per 100 000 live births between 1990 and 2015 [6].

The purpose of this paper is to review the available evidence regarding the effectiveness of CBPHC in improving maternal health broadly defined. It extends the focus of a previous review by Kidney et al. [7] that was limited to controlled studies of the effectiveness of community–level interventions in reducing maternal mortality. It also extends the findings of a recently published review by Lassi et al. (2016) [8] by providing a broader and more in–depth review of community–based approaches to improving maternal health.

This review is derived from assessments of projects, programs and research studies (hereafter referred to as projects) that implemented community–based interventions and measured their impact on maternal health. Our paper is part of a series on the effectiveness of CBPHC in improving maternal, neonatal and child health also reported in this journal [9–14].

METHODS

We conducted a search on PUBMED for assessments of CBPHC on maternal health. We defined such assessments of effectiveness broadly, as any document that assessed the effect of a CBPHC intervention on maternal health irrespective of inclusion of assessment of outcome on fetal, newborn or child health outcomes. The shared review methods for this series are described elsewhere in this series [9]. In addition, our maternal review searched additional databases including POPLINE, the Cochrane Review system, and CABI Publishing Database Subsets to identify additional documents. We included assessments identified from review articles. We made requests to knowledgeable professionals and organizations in the field of global public health for further listings of documents to be considered for inclusion. In order to provide a comprehensive set of documents that not only included clinical trials but also quasi–experimental designs, pre–post comparisons, program evaluations, and general descriptions of intervention effect, we used broad inclusion criteria.

Documents were eligible for inclusion in the present assessment if they: (1) involved an intervention intended to improve maternal health; (2) included interventions that took place outside of a health facility; (3) measured a change in maternal health (mortality, morbidity, nutritional status, or population coverage of a key maternal service) (eg, antenatal care attendance, facility–based delivery, attended delivery); (4) assessed an activity targeting a change in maternal health. We defined CBPHC, as a health intervention with a community component based outside of a physical health facility.

Two of the authors (HP, MJ) reviewed the abstracts of 7890 articles published on PUBMED through December 2015. Of these, 120 met criteria for inclusion. Additionally, 33 documents that were identified from the gray literature through searches of personal and colleague databases met criteria for inclusion. A total of 152 assessments met the final inclusion criteria. Two reviewers independently abstracted information from these assessments using a standardized data extraction form; a third independent reviewer resolved any discrepancies between the initial two reviews to provide a final summative review. The data were transferred to an electronic database and initially analyzed in EPI INFO version 3.5.4 (Epi Info, US Centers for Disease Control and

Prevention, Atlanta, Georgia, USA). Microsoft Excel (Microsoft, Seattle WA, USA) was used for additional descriptive analyses. Appendix S1 in **Online Supplementary Document** contains the references for these 152 assessments; the assessments and year cited in the main text in parentheses are followed by the letter "S" and a number indicating the order of the reference in Appendix S1 in **Online Supplementary Document**. In the tables, these assessments are cited by the first author and year followed in parentheses by the letter "S" and a number indicating the order of the reference in Appendix S1 in **Online Supplementary Document**.

Reviewers who extracted data defined outcome indicators as primary and secondary depending on the type of project and its goals. In general, primary outcomes had study designs that provided sufficient power to detect a statistically significant difference in that outcome, while assessments of secondary outcomes were not similarly powered. Here we describe the basic characteristics of the full database of maternal articles and present a more detailed descriptive analysis of documents from this database that measured the effects of interventions on the primary outcomes of maternal mortality and morbidity. We describe the key characteristics of the interventions employed by each project as well as the strength of evidence of effectiveness. We include descriptions of documents that failed to report significance or reported statistically insignificant effects to provide a fair representation of the field and to avoid only reporting positive results.

To more fully explore the impact of community–based interventions on maternal health outcomes, we make a brief description of changes in the population coverage of antenatal care, attended delivery, and facility–based delivery. However, including these in as detailed an assessment as we have conducted for primary mortality and morbidity outcomes will be reserved for a subsequent article.

RESULTS

Community settings

Bangladesh, India, Pakistan and Nepal were the location of the largest number of assessments (16, 15, 14 and 11, respectively). Data from a total of 169 countries were included in these 152 assessments. Six assessments included data from multiple countries in multiple regions. Countries were from six geographic regions, with the majority of them in South–East Asia (41%) and West Sub–Saharan Africa (22%). The majority of the 152 assessments were performed in rural communities (83%), with 11% in peri–urban and 10% in urban locations. The largest percentage (48%) of the 152 assessments were performed for an intervention that took place at the district or sub–province level; 8% took place at the province level; and 3% at the national level. 30% of interventions took place in a group of communities, and 9% took place in a single community.

Interventions

Each assessment described the effectiveness of one or more discrete interventions, ranging in number from 1 to 27. (A copy of the data extraction form is contained in Online Supplementary Document of another paper in this series [9]). As shown in **Figure 1**, a small number of assessments (2%) described the implementation of only one intervention; a majority (72%) of the documents described packages comprised of between 1 and 10 interventions.

In total, the 152 assessments described 1298 discrete interventions. 57% of these interventions promoted or provided routine maternal health care. These activities included antenatal and postpartum visits, immunizations, attendance of a skilled attendant at delivery, or making referrals to higher levels of care. 37% of these interventions addressed medical complications of pregnancy. These activities included screening and treating medical conditions such as high–risk pregnancy, gestational diabetes, hypertensive disorders, and infections. 6% of these interventions targeted socio–economic conditions of the

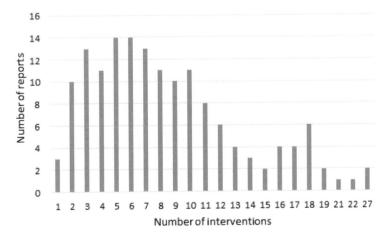

Figure 1. *Number of interventions implemented in individual assessments of the effectiveness of community-based primary health care in improving maternal health.*

mother, including participation in micro–credit and savings groups, conditional cash transfers, women's empowerment programs, and participatory
women's groups.

Box 1 describes three examples of intervention packages from three assessments with a larger number of kinds of interventions.

Box 1. *Examples of community–based intervention packages for improving maternal health*

Example 1. A community–based package implemented in 12 villages in rural In-
dia included the following interventions [15]:
- Provision of services at outreach sites by facility–based providers
- Provision of weekly antenatal clinics at outreach sites
- Provision of home visits for antenatal care by public health nurses
- Provision of treatment for simple illnesses by community health workers
- Provision of maternal education on child birth, child care, breastfeeding, immu-
  nizations, family spacing, and home economics by community health workers
- Distribution of iron/folate tablets in the community
- Identification of high–risk mothers in the community by community health
  workers and referral to a higher level of care

Example 2. A community–based package implemented in eight states in northern
India included the following interventions [16]:
- Provision of antenatal and postnatal home visits by health workers
- Provision of tetanus immunizations
- Provision/promotion of iron–folic acid tablets
- Behavior change messages to promote saving money for birth planning and
  childbirth;
- Promotion of delivery at a facility and, if a home delivery is planned, promo-
  tion of the use of a skilled birth attendant
- Promotion of immediate postpartum breastfeeding

Example 3. A package of community–based interventions implemented in four dis-
tricts of rural Bangladesh [17]:
- Formation of village health committees
- Training and linking traditional birth attendants to community health workers
- Promotion of family planning
- Identification of pregnancies at an early stage
- Promotion of birth planning
- Promotion of delivery by a trained health worker
- Promotion of immediate and exclusive breastfeeding
- Provision of antenatal care, delivery care, and postnatal care
- Promotion of vaccinations for pregnant women
- Referral for maternal complications
- Facilitate access to clinical services in health facilities

Categorization of outcome indicators

The 152 assessments described a multitude of outcome indicators. Categorization of outcome indicators aids in the assessment of intervention effectiveness. We extracted counts of indicators in five categories: (1) maternal mortality, (2) maternal morbidity, (3) population coverage of antenatal care attendance, (4) population coverage of deliveries by a skilled provider or a trained traditional birth attendant, and (5) population coverage of deliveries taking place at a facility. 19% of the assessments included maternal mortality as an indicator, and 21% measured maternal morbidity. In addition, 50% of the assessments measured antenatal care attendance; 66% measured attendance of deliveries by a skilled provider or trained traditional birth attendant; and 69% measured facility deliveries. A complete list of the outcome indicators among these 152 assessments is included in Online Supplementary Document of another article in this series [9].

Impact on maternal mortality

A maternal death was defined in the majority of assessments according to WHO definition: the death of a pregnant woman or a woman within 6 weeks of cessation of pregnancy, from any cause related to the pregnancy or its management, but excluding accidental causes. Of the 32 documents that assessed maternal mortality, 15 assessed mortality as a primary outcome indicator (**Table 1**). Of the 7 assessments that performed statistical significance testing, 6 reported significant decreases in mortality ranging from 42% to 78% and 1 suggested a trend toward increased mortality but this effect was not significant (**Table 1**). This suggestion of an increased mortality effect was only present when the facility–based intervention was analyzed together with the community arm, in comparison to the control arm. The suggestion of effect reversed in direction when the community arm was considered by itself against the control, with a 9% (non–significant) reduction in odds of maternal mortality rate (odds ratio OR 0.91, 95% confidence interval CI 0.51–1.63) (Colbourn 2013, reference [S39] in Appendix 1 in **Online Supplementary Document**). The design of the remaining 8 assessments with maternal mortality as a primary outcome did not permit statistical testing, but in all these assessments there was suggestion of decrease in maternal mortality. These reports suggested substantial impact, with four reporting a reduction to zero maternal deaths post–intervention (Asha–India 2008 [S19]; Curamericas Guatemala A&B 2007 [S41–42]; Lamb 1984 [S73]; Emond 2002 [S47]) and the remainder suggesting substantial decreases compared to regional or national population–level comparisons.

Table 1. *Effect size, direction and significance of community–based primary health care on maternal mortality outcomes**

Docu-ment	Intervention type	Effect	Study popula-tion	Effect size and confidence interval	Significance level†
Colbourn 2013 [S39]	Participatory women's groups in the community and quality improvement at health centers	Increase	Two–by–two factorial cluster randomized controlled trial of community compared to facility intervention, 14 576 births during baseline and 20 576 births during intervention, in 3 districts in rural Malawi, over 29 months from 2007–2010	8% increase in odds of maternal mortality in facility + community arm compared to control (OR: 1.08, 95% CI, 0.46–2.57)	$P = 0.854$
Manand-har 2004 [S83]	Participatory women's groups in the community, with 9 meetings per month and action–learning cycle	Decrease	Cluster–randomized controlled trial of 12 pairs of community clusters in 28 931 women in rural Nepal, over 2 years from 2001–2003	78% decrease in odds of maternal mortality in community intervention clusters compared to control clusters (OR: 0.22, 95% CI, 0.05–0.90), a maternal mortality ratio of 69 compared to 341 per 100 000 live births, respectively	**Significant, based on confidence interval** (*P* value not reported)
Zhenxu-an 1995 [S152]	Linked community–based mass health education campaign with facility– and community–based strengthening of emergency services	Decrease	Quasi–experimental pilot study compared to control area, covering 8000 deliveries per year in one county in peri–urban China, over 3 years from 1985–1988	Maternal mortality ratio (per 100 000 live births) decreased by 75.7% in the intervention areas and by 5.5% ($P > 0.05$) in the control areas	$P < 0.001$
Seim 2014 [S128]	Community mobilization to identify and refer protracted labor cases	Decrease	Pilot impact assessment, 12 254 births in rural Niger over 3 years from 2008–2011	Birth–related maternal mortality ratio fell by 73% over 3 y, from 630 to 170 per 100 000 live births	$P < 0.001$

Table 1. *Continued*

Document	Intervention type	Effect	Study population	Effect size and confidence interval	Significance level†
Koenig 1988 [S70]	Provision of community–based family planning services	Decrease	Quasi–experimental study compared intervention to control areas using demographic surveillance data from 187 523 people in 149 villages, 70 in intervention and 79 in control, in Matlab, Bangladesh over 9 years from 1976–1985	Significant overall decrease in maternal mortality rate for intervention vs control (66 vs 121 deaths per 100 000 women of childbearing age) but no significant change in maternal mortality ratio (effect size not reported)	P < 0.001
Fauveau 1991 [S51]	Provision of antenatal and maternity care and surveillance of vital events in the home and community	Decrease	Non–randomized evaluation of intervention villages compared to neighboring non– intervention villages with 196.000 total population, in rural Bangladesh over 3 years from 1978–1981	65% decrease in odds of maternal mortality in intervention compared to control area (OR: 0.35, 95% CI, 0.13–0.93), or 140 vs 380 per 100 000 live births	P < 0.05
Fauveau 1990 [S50]	Provision of primary and preventive care (maternal and child) in the home and community	Decrease	Non–randomized evaluation of intervention villages compared to neighboring non– intervention villages with 196 000 total population, in rural Bangladesh over 3 years from 1978–1981	42% lower rate of maternal mortality in control vs intervention (authors reported RR in control over intervention: RR 1.73, 95% CI, 1.02–2.93) (rate of 5.0 vs rate of 8.6 per 10 000 women of child–bearing age)	P < 0.05
Asha–India 2008 [S19]	Provision of community–based primary and antenatal care and women's empowerment in slum communities	Decrease	Program evaluation of intervention population of 300 000 people in urban slums in India, over 20 years, reporting data from 2007–2008	Zero deaths in Asha slums compared to 540 per 100 000 live births in India country– wide	N/A (maternal mortality ratio in slum areas compared to overall country ratio)

Table 1. *Continued*

Docu-ment	Intervention type	Effect	Study popula-tion	Effect size and confidence interval	Significance level†
CARE Nicaragua 2008 [S33]	Increase access and improve quality of maternal services through linking communities to facilities and through community mobilization and communication campaign	Decrease	Program evaluation of intervention in population of 174 367 (58 052 women of reproductive age) in 173 rural communities in Nicaragua over 5 years from 2002–2007	Maternal mortality rate decreased from 150 to 34 per 100 000 live births, with an annual average of 5500 deliveries over the 6 years of the intervention; maternal mortality ratio for the entire intervention area decreased from 119 to 60 per 100 000 live births over that time as well (a decrease of 49.2% compared to a national decrease of 42.6%)	N/A (maternal mortality rate decreased from baseline to endline in the primary referral hospital intervention area)
Curamericas–Guatemala–A&B 2007 [S41–42]	Care Groups and community–based impact–oriented care delivery/surveillance	Decrease	Program evaluation of intervention in population ranging in size from 11 123 (at end evaluation) to 14 272 (at mid-point) women of reproductive age, in 3 rural municipalities in Guatemala over 5 years from 2002–2007	Maternal mortality ratio decreased in all intervention areas relative to national data used as control (508 per 100 000 live births to zero, and 51124 per 100 000 live births to zero, over 4 years of data)	N/A (not powered sufficiently for statistical testing; diverse results)
Foord 1995 [S54]	Provision of primary and antenatal care in the community, and establishment of referral linkages	Decrease	Non–randomized evaluation of intervention compared to similar control area, each with a population of 1300, in a rural district of the Gambia over 2 years from 1989–1991	1 death in intervention area compared to 5 deaths in control area, giving a maternal mortality ratio of 130 per 100 000 live births in the intervention compared to 700 in control area	N/A (not powered sufficiently for statistical testing)

Table 1. *Continued*

Document	Intervention type	Effect	Study population	Effect size and confidence interval	Significance level†
Lamb 1984 [S73]	Provision of direct medical care, nutrition and vital statistics surveillance in community	Decrease	Non–randomized non–controlled evaluation of intervention impact in 4 villages with total population of 2000, in rural Gambia over 10 years from 1974–1984	No pregnancy–related deaths (per 1000 women of child bearing age) were observed in the community for the 8 years of intervention, compared to the annual 16 that would be expected using rates in comparable non–intervention areas	N/A (not powered sufficiently for statistical testing)
Emond 2002 [S47]	Provision of antenatal care in the community	Decrease	Non–randomized non–controlled evaluation of an intervention in a population of 42 000 in an urban district in Brazil over 30 months from 1995–1997	Maternal mortality ratio decreased from 335 per 100 000 live births prior to intervention, to zero maternal deaths during the 1 year after the intervention	N/A (not powered sufficiently for statistical testing)
Purdin 2009 [S117]	Community education campaign and creation of emergency obstetric centers linked to primary care centers	Decrease	Non–randomized non–controlled evaluation of intervention among community of 96 300 Afghan refugees in Pakistan over 4 years from 2004–2007	Annual maternal mortality ratio decreased from 291 to 102 per 100 000 live births over 4 years	N/A (baseline and endline rates calculated from two separate sources)
Findley 2015 [S53]	Behavior change and health systems integration	Decrease	Non–randomized evaluation of intervention compared to control and before compared to after, of 2360 women at baseline and 4628 at follow–up, in 3 states in northern Nigeria over 4 years from 2009–2013	Estimated maternal mortality ratio showed a larger decrease in the intervention than in the control communities, from 1270 to 1057 (interventions) and to 1262 (controls) per 100 000 live births	N/A (based on estimates)

N/A – not available; RR – rate ratio, CI – confidence interval, OR – odds ratio
* For assessments in which maternal mortality was the primary outcome indicator. The full references are shown in Appendix S1 in **Online Supplementary Document**.
† Significant results indicated in bold font.

Impact on maternal morbidity

29 of the 152 assessments measured changes in maternal morbidity, most commonly measuring postpartum hemorrhage (14 assessments), anemia (13), eclampsia (8) or malaria (6). Of these 29 documents that assessed maternal morbidity, 7 assessed a discrete morbidity as a primary outcome indicator and so are described in **Table 2**. Six of these assessments reported a significant decrease in at least one of the maternal morbidity indicators; one assessment suggested a decrease but did not report significance testing, and none reported a worsening of maternal morbidity.

Postpartum hemorrhage

Three of the seven documents measured change in postpartum hemorrhage following a preventive intervention delivered by a community health worker. These documents used the standard definition of measured blood loss greater than or equal to 500mL, and defined severe postpartum hemorrhage as blood loss greater than or equal to 1000mL (Kapungu 2013 [S65]; Fauveau 1990 [S50]; Derman 2006 [S45]). The three measurements of reduction in postpartum hemorrhage were statistically significant, with decreases ranging from 24% to 66% (**Table 2**). One assessment reported a significant decrease in severe postpartum hemorrhage, and the remaining two did not have a significant effect on severe postpartum hemorrhage.

Malaria

Two assessments reported measures of primary outcomes related to malaria, including the prevalence of anemia in malaria–endemic areas (two assessments) and the prevalence of maternal malarial episodes (one assessment). Of note, two of these assessments pertained to different aspects of a single intervention but were reported in separate peer–reviewed publications. One document reported equivalent, significant decreases in anemia in both community–based and facility–based intermittent preventive treatment (IPT) of malaria in pregnancy, (mean hemoglobin increased by 6.7% with 2 doses of IPT in both arms) (Mbonye 2008–5 [S90]). However, the women in the community arm received their first dose of IPT as recommended (during the second trimester) more frequently than the women in the facility arm (92.4% in the community vs 76.1% in the facility, $P < 0.001$). Women in the community arm also received IPT at a significantly earlier stage of pregnancy compared to those in the facility arm (21 weeks vs 23 weeks, $P < 0.001$), and the results described significant-

Table 2. *Effect size, direction and significance of community–based primary health care on maternal morbidity outcomes**

Refer-ence	Intervention type	Effect	Population	Effect size and confidence interval	Sig-nificance level†
Incidence of postpartum hemorrhage (PPH)					**PPH, Severe PPH‡**
Derman 2006 [S45]	Auxiliary nurse midwives (ANMs) administered oral misoprostol (or placebo) at home births they attended	Decrease	A randomized placebo–controlled trial assigned 812 women to oral misoprostol and 808 to placebo after home–based delivery by 25 ANMs, in rural India over 3 years from 2002–2005	47% decrease in incidence of PPH (6.4% in intervention vs 12.6% in control, RR: 0.53, 95% CI: 0.39–0.74); 83% decrease in severe PPH (0.2% in intervention vs 1.2% in control, RR: 0.16, 95% CI: 0.04–0.91). 1 case PPH prevented for every 18 women given chemoprophylaxis	PPH $P < 0.001$, severe PPH $P < 0.001$
Mobeen 2011 [S95]	Trained traditional birth attendants (TBAs) administered misoprostol (or placebo) at home deliveries they attended	Decrease	A randomized double–blind placebo-controlled trial assigned 534 women to oral misoprostol and 585 to placebo after home–based delivery by 81 TBAs, in one province in rural Pakistan over 24 months from 2006–2007	24% reduction in PPH after delivery (16.5% in intervention vs 21.9% in control, RR: 0.76, 95% CI 0.59–0.97); Insignificant decrease in severe PPH (RR: 0.57, 95% CI: 0.27–1.22)	PPH $P < 0.05$; NS
Stanton 2013 [S138]	Community health officers injected prophylactic oxytocin (or placebo) at home births they attended	Decrease	A community–based, cluster–randomized controlled trial assigned births conducted by 54 community health officers were randomized to study arm by officer, in 4 rural districts in Ghana, 689 in intervention and 897 in control, over 19 months from 2011–2012	Reduction of 51% in PPH (2.6% in intervention vs 5.5% in control, RR: 0.49, 95% CI: 0.27–0.88) No significant change in severe PPH (1 case in intervention, 8 in control group)	PPH $P < 0.05$; NS
Prevalence of malaria and anemia in malaria treatment interventions					
Mbonye 2008–5 [S90]	4 cadres of community health workers administered intermittent preventive treatment (IPT) for malaria in pregnancy in the community, compared to routine care in health clinics	Decrease	A non–randomized community trial assigned 2081 women (21 communities) to intervention and 704 women (4 communities) to control in 9 sub–counties of one district in central, rural Uganda over 21 months from 2003–2005	Prevalence of malaria episodes decreased from 49.5% to 17.6% in intervention and from 39.1% to 13.1% in control (both $P < 0.001$). 67.5% of women in the community–based intervention received IPT compared to 39.9% in facility–based control ($P < 0.001$)	$P < 0.001$; Significance for RR difference in reported malaria was not reported

Table 2. *Continued*

REFER-ENCE	INTERVENTION TYPE	EFFECT	POPULATION	EFFECT SIZE AND CONFIDENCE INTERVAL	SIG-NIFICANCE LEVEL†
Incidence of postpartum hemorrhage (PPH)					**PPH, Severe PPH‡**
Mbonye 2008–3 [S89]	4 cadres of community health workers administered intermittent preventive treatment for malaria in pregnancy in the community, compared to in health clinics	Decrease	A non–randomized community trial assigned 2081 women (21 communities) to intervention and 704 women (4 communities) to control in 9 sub–counties of one district in central, rural Uganda over 21 months from 2003–2005	Decreased prevalence of reported malaria episodes in both community and facility distribution of IPT (64% in community, from 49.5% to 17.6%, vs 66% decrease in facilities, from 39.1%, to 13.1%) (both *P* < 0.001)	*P* < 0.001 [Significance for RR difference in reported malaria was not reported]
Ndiaye 2009 [S105]	Positive deviance program using community–based volunteers to promote maternal health and nutrition, and to distribute iron supplements, to control anemia during pregnancy	Decrease (improvement)	A quasi–experimental design using pre–post evaluation of independent cross–section samples assessed 371 women in one community in rural Senegal over 9 months in 2003	75% reduction in risk of anemia, based on mean hemoglobin measurements, in the intervention compared to control area (no positive deviance) (OR: 0.25, 95% CI: 0.12–0.53)	*P* < 0.003§
Eclampsia					
Shamsuddin 2005 [S130]	Quasi–experimental study involving community, home–based administration of magnesium sulfate to diagnosed eclamptic and severe eclamptic cases prior to referral to hospital, compared to control cases who did not receive injections	Decrease	256 cases from 3 districts in Bangladesh, 133 in intervention and 132 in control, over 6 months in 2001	Decreased number of mean convulsions in the intervention cases (4.7 ± SD2.64) compared to control cases (6.86 ± SD 2.97) (*P* < 0.001)	*P* < 0.001

CI – confidence interval, SD – standard deviation, OR – odds ratio, PPH – postpartum hemorrhage, NS – not (statistically) significant, RR – rate ratio

*For assessments that analyzed maternal morbidity as a primary outcome indicator. The full references are shown in Appendix S1 in **Online Supplementary Document**.

†Significant results indicated in bold font.

‡PPH defined in each assessment as blood loss ≥500 mL; severe PPH defined in each assessment as blood loss ≥1000 mL.

§Chi–square test of difference between control and intervention.

ly higher adherence to the recommended two doses in the community arm compared to the facility arm. The community–based approach increased access to and use of IPT (Mbonye 2008–5, [S90]). The second assessment measured prevalence of reported malaria episodes and reported similar decreases in both community and facility distribution groups, but did not report significance testing of the relative difference in risk (Mbonye 2008–3 [S89]). One report assessed the prevalence of anemia, reporting a significant decrease of 75% in the intervention area vs the control area (Ndiaye 2009 [S105]).

Eclampsia

One assessment measured frequency of convulsions in eclamptic or pre–eclamptic cases who received magnesium sulfate injections at home prior to hospital transfer, reporting a significant decrease compared to cases who did not receive injections at home (Shamsuddin 2005, [S130]).

Impact on population coverage of evidence–based interventions

Antenatal care

Of the 37 assessments that measured coverage of antenatal attendance as a primary outcome indicator, 34 assessments reported increased attendance for antenatal care (ANC). No assessments observed a decrease in ANC coverage. Three assessments found no change in coverage, and we describe those three here in some detail.

The first assessment that found no change in ANC coverage (Helen Keller International 2003, [S60]) was an evaluation of a pilot program in Mozambique that provided iron and folic acid along with anemia–related health education to communities with a high anemia burden. Both recipient (intervention) and non–recipient (control) barrios showed some increases and some decreases on numerous outcome indicators such as knowledge of anemia, ingestion of iron/folic acid supplements, and reported anemia during most recent pregnancy.

The second assessment with no change in ANC attendance (More 2012 [S97]) was a cluster–randomized controlled trial testing the impact of creating and mobilizing women's groups in urban slums in Mumbai, India for the purpose of improving perinatal health, including increasing attendance at ANC clinics which had been strengthened through a city–wide maternal and newborn health care program for the urban poor. Although the assessment did report a reduction in the odds of a set of maternal morbidities in the intervention compared to control group (OR 0.60, 95% CI 0.38–0.94), there were no improvements in ANC attendance or other outcomes such as institutional delivery, breastfeeding, care–seeking, stillbirth rate, or neonatal mortality.

The third assessment that found no change in ANC coverage (Langston 2014, [S74]) was a mixed–methods evaluation of integrated community case management for childhood illness that was combined with promotion of maternal ANC attendance. ANC attendance increased in both control and intervention communities, but the difference was not statistically significant.

Changes in attended delivery

12 assessments measured coverage of the presence of a skilled or trained attendant at delivery as a primary outcome indicator. All 12 assessments reported an increase in the coverage of attended deliveries. The precise definition of a skilled or trained birth attendant varied among the assessments, and we have not attempted to standardize the definition here. Nine assessments specifically measured percentage of deliveries attended by a "skilled birth attendant," while one assessment measured the percentage of deliveries attended by a trained traditional birth attendant. Two assessments measured the attendance by a traditional birth attendant as compared to completely unattended deliveries. The two assessments that calculated the statistical significance of coverage changes found a significant increase.

Changes in facility–based deliveries

Eight assessments measured the percentage of births occurring in a facility as a primary outcome indicator. None of these assessments observed a decrease in coverage; one observed no change in coverage and seven reported an increase. The types of facilities included in these assessments were hospitals, health centers, and birthing huts.

Implementers

Community health workers (CHWs) were involved in intervention implementation in 132 of the 152 projects included in our database. In addition to CHWs, project implementers included local government health professionals (78/152 projects), local community members not trained as CHWs (48/152 projects), research staff hired specifically to implement the project (31/152 projects), and expatriates (4/152 projects). Multiple categories of implementers were present in three–fourths (71%) of the individual projects. CHWs were most frequently combined with local government health officials (69 assessments), and with non–CHW members of the local community (40 assessments).

Implementation strategies

Common strategies used to implement the interventions discussed above are highlighted here.

A typical set of implementation strategies is the following (Baqui 2008 [S24]):

- Used existing government ministry of health infrastructure (facilities and personnel)
- Combined maternal and newborn interventions
- Integrated nutrition with primary care services
- Delivered services and promoted interventions through both skilled and traditional health workers
- Used home visits and health centers to deliver interventions

Community–based strategies used to strengthen maternal health often over-lap with community–based strategies to improve neonatal and child health. Strategies to implement community–based interventions for improving neo-natal and child health are reported elsewhere [13]. These common strategies include:

- Established community collaborations such as the formation of commu-nity health committees
- Engaged community leaders to mobilize communities for a health–re-lated activity
- Formed community groups or collaborated with existing groups (includ-ing women's groups and micro–credit savings groups)
- Engaged communities in the selection and support of CHWs
- Engaged communities in the planning and/or evaluation of CBPHC pro-gramming

Home visits were a common strategy used to identify pregnant women, to provide health services and education/counseling, as well as to promote healthy behaviors such as family planning and facility delivery. Home visits were also used to provide postpartum maternal care and identify postpartum mothers with problems requiring referral. The formation and strengthening of participatory women's groups was a common strategy to motivate women and their families to seek antenatal, delivery and emergency obstetrical care.

Outreach visits to the community by a mobile health team based at a peripheral health facility were also a common approach to provide prenatal care, family planning services, and maternal immunizations.

Community–based approaches, particularly through home visits provided by CHWs, are commonly used to increase the coverage of insecticide–treated bed nets for pregnant women and to expand the coverage of intermittent preventive treatment of malaria in malaria–endemic areas. These are interventions that are effective not only for improving maternal outcomes but also for improving perinatal and neonatal outcomes. Community–based approaches to expand the detection of women with HIV infection and to increase the coverage of anti–retroviral treatment of HIV–positive pregnant women include CHWs making home visits and mobile outreach teams.

Health systems strengthening strategies associated with CBPHC for improving maternal health include facilitating referrals (by forming community emergency response committees, community transport systems, and community savings or insurance schemes to cover transport and hospital costs when obstetric emergencies arise). Other health–system–related activities often carried out by projects that also implemented CBPHC interventions included strengthening the quality of care provided at peripheral health facilities (by improving logistics and training staff), and strengthening the supervisory system of community–level workers.

DISCUSSION

This analysis provides evidence for a positive impact of CBPHC interventions on reducing maternal morbidity, increasing population coverage of evidence–based interventions, and possibly contributing to reductions in maternal mortality in selected settings. Six of the seven assessments that were able to measure the statistical significance of the change in maternal mortality showed a statistically significant decrease. There were eight additional assessments that reported trends in maternal mortality but could not measure the statistical significance of the impact. All eight of these reported a favorable effect on maternal mortality. In contrast to a 2010 Cochrane review of the impact of community–based interventions, which reported reductions in maternal morbidity but no reduction in maternal mortality [18], our inclusion criteria were broad and allowed non–randomized assessments as well as assessments from the gray literature.

All three assessments of the statistical significance of impact of CBPHC interventions on the incidence of postpartum hemorrhage showed significant decreases. One of the three showed a significant decrease in the incidence of severe postpartum hemorrhage (which was a secondary outcome for all three projects). Three assessments of CBPHC interventions on maternal malaria and malaria–related anemia all showed significant positive effects, and one assessment of CBPHC interventions on eclampsia showed a significant positive effect.

Our analysis of the effectiveness of CBPHC approaches in increasing the population coverage of evidence–based interventions focused on three interventions: antenatal care attendance, delivery trained provider, and facility–based delivery. Global recommendations for attendance at antenatal care have evolved over time to support increased contacts [19], and the provision of antenatal care as a community–based intervention may help to expand the coverage of more frequent, high–quality and woman–centered pregnancy care in resource–constrained settings.

Delivery attended by a skilled provider improves delivery outcomes [20], but delivery by a fully and formally trained midwife or other highly skilled provider is often beyond the short–term capacity of many countries for all births. Strategies that integrate both skilled and traditional birth attendants into the health system are important to increase skilled birth attendance [21,22]. Delivery at a health facility improves access to emergency and critical care for prompt attention to life–threatening maternal complications [3], although the literature points out deficiencies in quality that are commonly observed at facilities [2] and some argue that facility delivery is not a necessary requisite for the reduction of maternal mortality [23,24]. Despite these observations, promoting facility deliveries has been a focus of many interventions aimed at reaching the 2015 Millennium Development Goals for maternal health [25] and now for reaching the 2030 Sustainable Development Goals. However, recent literature suggests that a high rate of institutional delivery by itself is insufficient to reduce maternal mortality ratios [1,26].

A large proportion of the low–income populations globally live more than one hour away from a health facility [4], making utilization of health facilities and emergency care services a challenge. Therefore it is important to strengthen community–based interventions to promote antenatal care attendance, attended delivery, and facility delivery.

The vast majority of community–based primary care interventions described by assessments included in this study were implemented by a wide variety of different types of community–based health workers. It is important to continue efforts to incorporate them in the maternal care process as well as traditional birth attendants, who can serve as doulas (birth companions for facility births) and collaborators in the delivery [27]. Community–based interventions show great potential for reducing morbidity of mothers from malaria and hemorrhage following home delivery.

Study limitations

Maternal mortality is a rare event, even in settings where maternal mortality is relatively high: even with a maternal mortality ratio of 1000, only 1% of live births are associated with a maternal death. Thus, the demonstration of a statistically significant decline in maternal mortality is a challenge for field programs. As our findings indicate, there are numerous assessments in which there is a suggestion of maternal mortality impact, but the decline does not reach statistical significance. Additionally, there are examples in the literature in which the same community–based intervention shows a statistically significant reduction in maternal mortality in one setting [28] but not in another [29]. One of the explanations for this finding is that the study that did not show a statistically significant change was not adequately powered (meaning that an impact may have been achieved in reality but due to the small sample size it did not reach statistical significance).

This review did not focus on assessments of cost–effectiveness. It is worth noting that studies of the cost–effectiveness of community–based approaches to improving maternal health are rare. Additionally, it is important to note that there are certain settings in which CBPHC may not be effective in improving maternal health – for example in settings where high–quality facility–based care is available and utilized and therefore levels of maternal health are already high. Thus, the cost–effectiveness of CPBHC may be highly dependent on the context. Although evidence of the cost–effectiveness of community–based approaches for improving neonatal and child health care has been summarized [8], there is a need for more research on the cost–effectiveness of community–based maternal health interventions.

The local context in which the assessments were carried out is important to more fully understand which CBPHC components are most useful in which setting. The availability of trained personnel to provide maternity care, the availability and utilization of health facilities, and the local geographic context are all important in assessing how CBPHC can most effectively contribute to improve maternal health. However, to adequately explore these issues is beyond the scope of this paper.

This review did not assess the effects of community–based family planning interventions on maternal health because their effects are indirect and not readily measured in specific program settings, including in the assessments included in our review. However, there is extensive evidence that family planning is important for improving maternal health (by, among other things, reducing the number of maternal deaths simply by reducing the number of women who become pregnant). There is extensive evidence that family planning can be effectively provided through a community–based primary health care platform [30–32]. Had assessments of the effectiveness of community–based family planning been included in our review, we expect that the evidence for the effectiveness of CBPHC in improving maternal health would have been even more compelling.

Our inclusion of a wide variety of intervention packages precludes us from being able to make specific recommendations for or against intervention components in community–based approaches. However, other authors have summarized potential frameworks to select appropriate intervention package components [33,34]. The nature of intervention packages evolves with technology and with the emergence of new interventions. For example, mhealth strategies involving community health workers and women of reproductive age have the potential to link clients with services and promote utilization of services [35]. However, no studies assessing mHealth interventions were identified for our review. In addition, the lack of standardization of indicator measurement limits our ability to draw detailed conclusions. Finally, the richness of this data set is such that only a limited analysis of the data is provided here. Further analyses are needed, as pointed out at several points in this paper.

CONCLUSIONS

The evidence provided here supports the recommendation that CBPHC is an important component of a comprehensively–designed maternal health program – not only because of the direct effects it can have on reducing maternal morbidity and its potential to contribute to reductions in maternal mortality, but also because of its contributions to the promotion of appropriate facility utilization for ANC, childbirth, and referral of obstetrical emergencies. Finally, the closely related contributions that CBPHC can make to improving neonatal health are important as well but summarized in another article in this series [10].

Acknowledgments: We are grateful to the following organizations that provided small grants to cover the expenses of this review: UNICEF, the World Bank, the Department of Child and Adolescent Health and Development of the World Health Organization, the CORE Group (Collaboration and Resources for Child Health)/USAID, Future Generations, *and the Gates Foundation. We are also grateful to the American Public Health Association and particularly its International Health Section staff, which administered some of these funds. We thank Future Generations for providing office space, administrative support, and salary support to Dr Perry during the initial phase of the review. The World Bank made it possible for one of its consultants, Dr Bahie Rassekh, to participate as a member of the Study Team.*

Funding: *The following organizations provided funds that were used to conduct the work described in this article: The World Health Organization, UNICEF, the World Bank, the United States Agency for International Development, and the Gates Foundation. The organizations that provided financial support had no role in the execution of the review.*

Authorship contributions: *MJ wrote the first draft. MJ, SP and MS collected the evidence for this review and guided its analysis. All of the authors participated in the revision of earlier drafts and approved the final draft.*

Competing interests: *All authors have completed the Unified Competing Interest Form at www.icmje.org/coi_disclosure.pdf (available upon request from the corresponding author), and declare no conflict of interest.*

References

1 Randive B, Diwan V, De Costa A. India's Conditional Cash Transfer Programme (the JSY) to promote institutional Birth: is there an association between institutional birth proportion and maternal mortality? PLoS One. 2013;8:e67452. Medline:23826302 doi:10.1371/journal.pone.0067452

2 Hulton LA, Matthews Z, Stones RW. Applying a framework for assessing the quality of maternal health services in urban India. Soc Sci Med. 2007;64:2083-95. Medline:17374551 doi:10.1016/j.socscimed.2007.01.019

3 Kayongo M, Rubardt M, Butera J, Abdullah M, Mboninyibuka D, Madili M. Making EmOC a reality–CARE's experiences in areas of high maternal mortality in Africa. Int J Gynaecol Obstet. 2006;92:308-19. Medline:16442536 doi:10.1016/j.ijgo.2005.12.003

4 Pearson L, Shoo R. Availability and use of emergency obstetric services: Kenya, Rwanda, Southern Sudan, and Uganda. Int J Gynaecol Obstet. 2005;88:208-15. Medline:15694109 doi:10.1016/j.ijgo.2004.09.027

5 WHO, World Bank, UNICEF, UNFPA. Trends in Maternal Mortality: 1990 to 2015. 2015. Available: http://www.who.int/reproductivehealth/publications/monitoring/maternal-mortality-2015/en/. Accessed: 26 April 2017.

6 Alkema L, Chou D, Hogan D, Zhang S, Moller AB, Gemmill A, et al. Global, regional, and national levels and trends in maternal mortality between 1990 and 2015, with scenario-based projections to 2030: a systematic analysis by the UN Maternal Mortality Estimation Inter-Agency Group. Lancet. 2016;387:462-74. Medline:26584737 doi:10.1016/S0140-6736(15)00838-7

7 Kidney E, Winter HR, Khan KS, Gulmezoglu AM, Meads CA, Deeks JJ, et al. Systematic review of effect of community-level interventions to reduce maternal mortality. BMC Pregnancy Childbirth. 2009;9:2. Medline:19154588 doi:10.1186/1471-2393-9-2

8   Lassi ZS, Kumar R, Bhutta ZA. Community-based care to improve maternal, newborn, and child health. 2016. In: Disease Control Priorities: Reproductive, Maternal, Newborn, and Child Health, Third Edition [Internet]. Washington, DC: World Bank; [263-94]. Available: https://openknowledge.worldbank.org/bitstream/handle/10986/23833/9781464803482.pdf?sequence=3. Accessed: 26 April 2017.

9   Perry H, Rassekh B, Gupta S, Wilhelm J, Freeman P. A comprehensive review of the evidence regarding the effectiveness of community-based primary health care in improving maternal, neonatal and child health: 1. rationale, methods and database description. J Glob Health. 2017;7:010901.

10 Sacks E, Freeman P, Sakyi K, Jennings M, Rassekh B, Gupta S, et al. A comprehensive review of the evidence regarding the effectiveness of community-based primary health care in improving maternal, neonatal and child health: 3. neonatal health findings. J Glob Health. 2017;7:010903.

11 Freeman P, Schleiff M, Sacks E, Rassekh B, Gupta S, Perry H. A comprehensive review of the evidence regarding the effectiveness of community-based primary health care in improving maternal, neonatal and child health: 4. child health findings. J Glob Health. 2017;7:010904.

12 Schleiff M, Kumapley R, Freeman P, Gupta S, Rassekh B, Perry H. A comprehensive review of the evidence regarding the effectiveness of community-based primary health care in improving maternal, neonatal and child health: 5. equity effects. J Glob Health. 2017;7:010905.

13 Perry H, Rassekh B, Gupta S, Freeman P. A comprehensive review of the evidence regarding the effectiveness of community-based primary health care in improving maternal, neonatal and child health: 6. strategies used by effective projects. J Glob Health. 2017;7:010906.

14 Perry H, Rassekh B, Gupta S, Freeman P. A comprehensive review of the evidence regarding the effectiveness of community-based primary health care in improving maternal, neonatal and child health: 7. programs with evidence of long-term impact on mortality in children younger than five years of age. J Glob Health. 2017;7:010309.

15 Dutt D, Srinivasa DK. Impact of maternal and child health strategy on child survival in a rural community of Pondicherry. Indian Pediatr. 1997;34:785-92. Medline:9492416

16 Baqui A, Williams EK, Rosecrans AM, Agrawal PK, Ahmed S, Darmstadt GL, et al. Impact of an integrated nutrition and health programme on neonatal mortality in rural northern India. Bull World Health Organ. 2008;86:796-804. Medline:18949217 doi:10.2471/BLT.07.042226

17 Rahman M, Jhohura FT, Mistry SK, Chowdhury TR, Ishaque T, Shah R, et al. Assessing Community Based Improved Maternal Neonatal Child Survival (IMNCS) Program in Rural Bangladesh. PLoS One. 2015;10:e0136898. Medline:26340672 doi:10.1371/journal.pone.0136898

18 Lassi ZS, Haider BA, Bhutta ZA. Community-based intervention packages for reducing maternal and neonatal morbidity and mortality and improving neonatal outcomes. Cochrane Database Syst Rev. 2010;11:CD007754. Medline:21069697

19 WHO. Antenatal care in developing countries. Promises, achievements and missed opportunities: an analysis of trends, levels and differentials. 2003. Available: http://www.who.int/reproductivehealth/publications/maternal_perinatal_health/9241590947/en/. Accessed: 26 April 2017.

20 Homer CS, Friberg IK, Dias MA, ten Hoope-Bender P, Sandall J, Speciale AM, et al. The projected effect of scaling up midwifery. Lancet. 2014;384:1146-57. Medline:24965814 doi:10.1016/S0140-6736(14)60790-X

21 Byrne A, Morgan A. How the integration of traditional birth attendants with formal health systems can increase skilled birth attendance. Int J Gynaecol Obstet. 2011;115:127-34. Medline:21924419 doi:10.1016/j.ijgo.2011.06.019

22 Lane K, Garrod J. The return of the Traditional Birth Attendant. J Glob Health. 2016;6:020302. Medline:27606054 doi:10.7189/jogh.06.020302

23 Costello A, Azad K, Barnett S. An alternative strategy to reduce maternal mortality. Lancet. 2006;368:1477-9. Medline:17071268 doi:10.1016/S0140-6736(06)69388-4

24 Miller S, Cordero M, Coleman AL, Figueroa J, Brito-Anderson S, Dabagh R, et al. Quality of care in institutionalized deliveries: the paradox of the Dominican Republic. Int J Gynaecol Obstet. 2003;82:89-103, discussion 87-8. Medline:12834953 doi:10.1016/S0020-7292(03)00148-6

25 WHO. The World Health Report 2005 - make every mother and child count. 2005. Available: http://www.who.int/whr/2005/whr2005_en.pdf?ua=1. Accessed: 26 April 2017.

26 Souza JP, Gulmezoglu AM, Vogel J, Carroli G, Lumbiganon P, Qureshi Z, et al. Moving beyond essential interventions for reduction of maternal mortality (the WHO Multi-country Survey on Maternal and Newborn Health): a cross-sectional study. Lancet. 2013;381:1747-55. Medline:23683641 doi:10.1016/S0140-6736(13)60686-8

27 Stollak I, Valdez M, Rivas K, Perry H. Casas Maternas in the Rural Highlands of Guatemala: A Mixed-Methods Case Study of the Introduction and Utilization of Birthing Facilities by an Indigenous Population. Glob Health Sci Pract. 2016;4:114-31. Medline:27016548 doi:10.9745/GHSP-D-15-00266

28 Manandhar DS, Osrin D, Shrestha BP, Mesko N, Morrison J, Tumbahangphe KM, et al. Effect of a participatory intervention with women's groups on birth outcomes in Nepal: cluster-randomised controlled trial. Lancet. 2004;364:970-9. Medline:15364188 doi:10.1016/S0140-6736(04)17021-9

29 Azad K, Barnett S, Banerjee B, Shaha S, Khan K, Rego AR, et al. Effect of scaling up women's groups on birth outcomes in three rural districts in Bangladesh: a cluster-randomised controlled trial. Lancet. 2010;375:1193-202. Medline:20207412 doi:10.1016/S0140-6736(10)60142-0

30 Singh S, Darroch J, Ashford L. Adding It Up: The Costs and Benefits of Investing in Sexual and Reproductive Health 2014. 2014. Available: https://www.guttmacher.org/sites/default/files/report_pdf/addingitup2014.pdf. Accessed. 26 April 2017.

31 Prata N, Vahidnia F, Potts M, Dries-Daffner I. Revisiting community-based distribution programs: are they still needed? Contraception. 2005;72:402-7. Medline:16307960 doi:10.1016/j.contraception.2005.06.059

32 Stanback J, Spieler J, Shah I, Finger WR. Community-based health workers can safely and effectively administer injectable contraceptives: conclusions from a technical consultation. Contraception. 2010;81:181-4. Medline:20159172 doi:10.1016/j.contraception.2009.10.006

33 Kearns AD, Caglia JM, Ten Hoope-Bender P, Langer A. Antenatal and postnatal care: a review of innovative models for improving availability, accessibility, acceptability and quality of services in low-resource settings. BJOG. 2016;123:540-8. Medline:26694075 doi:10.1111/1471-0528.13818

34 Lunze K, Higgins-Steele A, Simen-Kapeu A, Vesel L, Kim J, Dickson K. Innovative approaches for improving maternal and newborn health–a landscape analysis. BMC Pregnancy Childbirth. 2015;15:337. Medline:26679709 doi:10.1186/s12884-015-0784-9

35 Labrique AB, Vasudevan L, Kochi E, Fabricant R, Mehl G. mHealth innovations as health system strengthening tools: 12 common applications and a visual framework. Glob Health Sci Pract. 2013;1:160-71. Medline:25276529 doi:10.9745/GHSP-D-13-00031

Acknowledgement: *originally published as: Mary Carol Jennings, Subarna Pradhan, Meike Schleiff, Emma Sacks, Paul A Freeman, Sundeep Gupta, Bahie M Rassekh, Henry B Perry:Comprehensive review of the evidence regarding the effectiveness of Community–Based Primary Health Care in improving maternal, neonatal and child health: 2. maternal health findings. Reprinted with permission from Edinburgh University Global Health Society under Creative Commons Attribution Licence (Journal of Global Health 2017; 010902).*

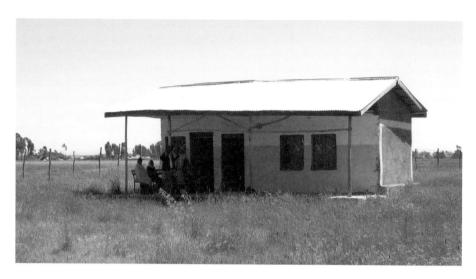

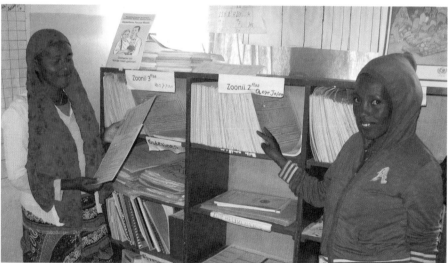

A health post and two Health Extension Workers with their family health folders. Each health post serves 5,000 people, and the Health Extension Workers spend half their time visiting homes in the community

Photocredit: Henry Perry (used with permission).

Comprehensive review of the evidence regarding the effectiveness of community–based primary health care in improving maternal, neonatal and child health: 3. neonatal health findings

Emma Sacks[1], Paul A Freeman[2,3], Kwame Sakyi[1], Mary Carol Jennings[1], Bahie M Rassekh[4], Sundeep Gupta[5], Henry B Perry[1]

[1] Department of International Health, Johns Hopkins Bloomberg School of Public Health, Baltimore, Maryland, USA
[2] Independent Consultant, Seattle, Washington, USA
[3] Department of Global Health, University of Washington, Seattle, Washington, USA
[4] The World Bank, Washington, District of Columbia, USA
[5] Medical Epidemiologist, Lusaka, Zambia

Background As the number of deaths among children younger than 5 years of age continues to decline globally through programs to address the health of older infants, neonatal mortality is becoming an increasingly large proportion of under–5 deaths. Lack of access to safe delivery care, emergency obstetric care and postnatal care continue to be challenges for reducing neonatal mortality. This article reviews the available evidence regarding the effectiveness of community–based primary health care (CBPHC) and common components of programs aiming to improve health during the first 28 days of life.

Methods A database comprising evidence of the effectiveness of projects, programs and field research studies (referred to collectively as projects) in improving maternal, neonatal and child health through CBPHC has been assembled and described elsewhere in this series. From this larger database (N = 548), a subset was created from assessments specifically relating to newborn health (N = 93). Assessments were excluded if the primary project beneficiaries were more than 28 days of age, or if the assessment did not identify one of the following outcomes related to neonatal health: changes in knowledge about newborn illness, care seeking for newborn illness, utilization of postnatal care, nutritional status of neonates, neonatal morbidity, or neonatal mortality. Descriptive analyses were conducted based on study type and outcome variables. An equity assessment was also conducted on the articles included in the neonatal subset.

Results There is strong evidence that CBPHC can be effective in improving neonatal health, and we present information about the common characteristics shared by effective programs. For projects that reported on health outcomes, twice as many reported an improvement in neonatal health as did those that reported no effect; only one study demonstrated a negative effect. Of those with the strongest experimental study design, almost three–quarters reported beneficial neonatal health outcomes. Many of the neonatal projects assessed in our database utilized community health workers (CHWs), home visits, and participatory women's groups. Several of the interventions used in these projects focused on health education (recognition of danger signs), and promotion of and support for exclusive breastfeeding (sometimes, but not always, including early breastfeeding). Almost all of the assessments that included a measurable equity component showed that CBPHC produced neonatal health benefits that favored the poorest segment of the project population. However, the studies were quite biased in geographic scope, with more than half conducted in South Asia, and many were pilot studies, rather than projects at scale.

Conclusions CBPHC can be effectively employed to improve neonatal health in high–mortality, resource–constrained settings. CBPHC is especially important for education and support for pregnant and postpartum mothers and for establishing community–facility linkages to facilitate referrals for obstetrical emergencies; however, the latter will only produce better health outcomes if facilities offer timely, high–quality care. Further research on this topic is needed in Africa and Latin America, as well as in urban and peri–urban areas. Additionally, more assessments are needed of integrated packages of neonatal interventions and of programs at scale.

Despite marked reductions in overall child mortality globally since 1990, 2.7 million live–born infants still die annually during their first month of life [1]. Neonatal mortality is becoming an increasingly large proportion of mortality among children younger than 5 years of age, at present accounting for 45% of under–5 deaths [2]. Approximately 73% of neonatal deaths occur during the first week of life [3], 36% on the first day of life [3] and 32% during the first 6 hours of life [4]. The key causes of death among neonates are complications of preterm birth, intrapartum–related complications (often birth asphyxia), and infections [5]. Given that 51% of births in the least developed countries, 49% of births in sub–Saharan Africa, and 41% of births in South Asia still take place outside of health facilities [1], and the continuing challenges with providing high–quality care in facilities, community–based approaches to improve neonatal health will be essential for the near term to promote healthy home practices and to reach newborns during their birth and soon thereafter when they have a high risk of mortality. Community–based efforts in education, support and referral may be important in settings with high facility delivery rates as well.

Community–based approaches to reducing neonatal mortality are of particular importance in low–income settings where home deliveries are common and access to facility–based care for neonates is limited [2,6,7]. This paper analyzes the findings related to the effectiveness of community–based primary health care (CBPHC) in improving neonatal health using a subset of articles from a database assembled for a broader review of the effectiveness of community–based primary health (CBPHC) in improving child health. It complements other reviews that have been carried out on this topic [7–9]. Projects were assessed by their study design, outcome variables, program components, and reported neonatal health impact.

METHODS

The methodology for assembling a database of 548 assessments of the effectiveness of CBPHC in improving child health, including the search strategy, has been described elsewhere in this series [10]. In brief, we considered CBPHC to be any activity in which one or more health–related interventions were carried out in the community outside of a health facility. There could also be associated activities that took place in health facilities. The larger study conducted a search of published documents in PubMed, personal sources, and the grey literature for documents that described the implementation of CBPHC and assessed the effect of these projects, programs, or field research studies (described collectively as projects) on mortality, morbidity, nutritional status, or population coverage of an evidence–based intervention. Of 4276 articles identified for screening via PubMed, 433 qualified for the review. In addition, 115 reports were identified from the grey literature and elsewhere, yielding a total of 548 neonatal and child health assessments included in the review. Two reviewers independently extracted information about the assessment and a third independent reviewer resolved any differences. The data were transferred to an electronic database using EPI INFO version 3.5.4 (US Centers for Disease Control and Prevention, Atlanta, Georgia, USA).

Starting with the child health data set, assessments were selected for the analysis of neonatal health in a three–stage process (**Figure 1**). In the first stage, articles were selected that had been coded with relevant interventions pertaining to neonates. These interventions, as defined on the data extraction form, were: neonatal/perinatal health; breastfeeding; child weight/height (including birth weight); immunizations; diarrhea treatment; pneumonia treatment; malaria prevention; malaria treatment; Integrated Management of Childhood Illness (IMCI); prevention of mother–to–child transmission of HIV; neonatal tetanus prevention; neonatal tetanus treatment; congenital syphilis prevention; congenital syphilis treatment; and primary health care. This yielded 380 articles.

In the second stage, titles and abstracts of these 380 articles were reviewed.

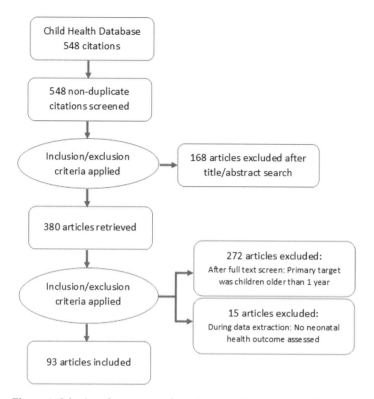

Figure 1. *Selection of assessments for inclusion in the neonatal health review.*

Articles were then excluded if the target population was not infants under age one. This yielded 108 articles. Further exclusions were made if the article did not have an outcome directly related to neonatal health (knowledge about newborn illness, care seeking for newborn illness, utilization of postnatal care, or a neonatal health outcome related to nutritional status, morbidity or mortality). The final database for this sub–analysis included 93 articles. Articles were coded by the primary and secondary health condition addressed, the outcome variables, and categorized by the type and strength of study design.

All study designs were included, but were separated into three categories: randomized controlled trials (RCTs); non–randomized controlled trials; and observational and other non–experimental designs. We conducted descriptive analyses on the data set to present the proportion of beneficial health outcomes within each category. A table of only the RCTs is presented in Table S1 of **Online Supplementary Document**.

In this paper, when assessments selected for this analysis are specifically cited, we cite them with the first author's last name and year of publication, with the reference number in brackets with a prefix S. The full reference can be obtained from Appendix S2 in **Online Supplementary Document** where the full references for all the 93 assessments selected for the analysis in this paper can be located.

The term community health worker (CHW) is used here to refer to any community–level actor who receives training from the project or the broader health system/health program to assist in the activities of the project. We do not provide any further specification here regarding length of training, level of compensation (if any), formal recognition by the ministry of health, or other descriptive characteristics of CHWs, as they varied widely among the included assessments, although we recognize that this is an important dimension of these projects.

RESULTS

Description of database

As shown in **Figure 2**, South Asia was far more represented than Africa or Latin America for assessments of the effectiveness of CBPHC in improving neonatal health. The country with the most reported assessments was India (with 16), followed by Bangladesh (12), Nepal (12) and Pakistan (6). Brazil

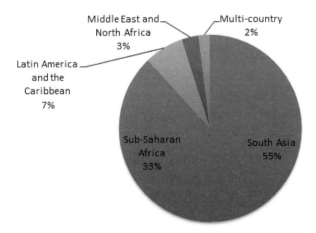

Figure 2. *Regions of the world where projects were implemented whose assessments are in the neonatal database (n = 93).*

had 4 assessments; Ghana, Kenya, Tanzania and Uganda, each had 3. Two assessments were of projects in more than one country: one implemented in 10 African countries and one in four countries in sub–Saharan Africa and South Asia.

Most of the 93 assessments in our analysis were of projects that focused on a set of communities (n = 36) or a district (n = 42). Very few studies (n = 10) were at the provincial, national or multinational level, and 5 projects were implemented in one community only. Overwhelmingly, the projects were in rural areas (n = 67), although some were in urban (n = 19) or peri–urban areas (n = 7). Projects were mostly implemented by CHWs (n = 61), and many utilized ministry of health staff (n = 37), local field researchers (n = 26) and local community members (n = 27); these categories were not mutually exclusive and there are many projects using paid or volunteer CHWs who were a formal part of ministry of health services.

Interventions implemented

Three–quarters (76%) of the 93 assessments identified for this review described projects that implemented what were classified in the data extraction process as "neonatal/perinatal health" interventions. Almost one–third of the assessments (38%) described a breastfeeding intervention, and one–quarter (24%) described an intervention that focused on the prevention of low birth weight or the care of low–birth weight infants. Other common activities carried out by these projects included general primary health care, immunizations, micronutrient distribution, malaria prevention or treatment, tetanus prevention, pneumonia treatment, and tetanus prevention; no studies addressed pneumonia prevention or tetanus treatment (**Table 1**).

Projects were generally implemented over a relatively short timeline. One–quarter (24%) of the assessments were implemented for less than one year, and another three–quarters (72%) were implemented for between one to five years. Fewer than 5% of the projects in the review were implemented for more than five years.

Outcomes

The assessments utilized a range of methodologies. Almost half (46%) were randomized controlled trials (RCTs), and another 15% were quasi–experimental (non–randomized, controlled) trials. A fifth of the projects (21%) used an uncontrolled before–after study design, and a tenth (9%) used a descriptive

Table 1. *Interventions reported in assessments of community–based primary health care in improving neonatal health*

INTERVENTION	NUMBER OF ASSESSMENTS IN REVIEW*	PERCENTAGE (N = 93)
General promotion of improved neonatal health	67	72.0
Promotion of breastfeeding during the neonatal period	33	35.5
Promotion of improved weight among neonates (including birth weight)	21	22.6
Primary health care	15	16.1
Integrated Management of Childhood Illness (IMCI)	14	15.1
Diarrhea treatment	12	12.9
Malaria treatment	12	12.9
Immunizations	11	11.8
Malaria prevention	7	7.5
Neonatal tetanus prevention	7	7.5
Pneumonia treatment	7	7.5
HIV/AIDS (prevention of mother–to–child transmission of HIV)	5	5.4
Congenital syphilis prevention	1	1.1
Congenital syphilis treatment	1	1.1

*The column sums to more than 93 since many assessments described multiple interventions.

study design. Other study designs less commonly used were case–control and cross–sectional studies. Table S1 in **Online Supplementary Document** provides a summary of the RCT assessments.

Among the 93 assessments included in our analysis, 45 separate indicators were measured. **Table 2** and **Table 3** list these and classify them in terms of the Donabedian scheme [11] of input, process, output, outcome and impact indicators and also in terms of the type of outcome. Outcomes were classified as either: (1) a significant positive effect, or (2) no significant effect or (3) a significant negative effect. Positive or negative effects were all statistically significant ($P \leq 0.05$). No significant effects were those in which statistical testing demonstrated a difference that was not statistically significant ($P > 0.05$), or significance testing was not performed. **Table 2** and **Table 3** provide an analysis of effectiveness in terms of one or more of the types of health indicators that were used in selecting assessments for inclusion in the review by specific health outcome or process/output indicator. A few process/output indicators shown in **Table 3** did not meet the criteria for inclusion in the review (eg, knowledge measures, quality of care measures, care seeking for neonatal illness, participation in group activities, or birth preparedness) but they were measured as part of project assessments along with other health outcome indicators that did qualify, so we have included them in **Table 3**.

Table 2. *Assessments of community–based primary health care projects that document improvements in neonatal health as defined by health outcome and health impact indicators**

OUTCOME MEASURE	ASSESSMENT METHODOLOGY WITH FINDINGS						TOTAL
	Randomized controlled assessments		Non-randomized controlled assessments		Observational (mostly pre/post intervention) assessments		
	Positive effect (n = 31)	No significant or negative effect (n = 12)	Positive effect (n = 8)	No significant or negative effect (n = 2)	Positive effect (n = 13)	No significant or negative effect (n = 7)	
Nutritional status:							
Birth weight/low birth weight	Christian 2003 [S23]	Larocque 2006 [S46]				Ahrari 2006 [S2]; Tielsch 2008 [S82]	4
Small-for-gestational age	Christian 2003 [S23]						1
Preterm birth	Christian 2003 [S23]						1
Morbidity:							
Neonatal sepsis	Gill 2014 [S34]; Soofi 2012 [S77]						2
Neonatal omphalitis	Mullany 2006 [S53]; Soofi 2012 [S77]						2
HIV mother–to–child transmission/infection rate					Gupta 2013 [S36]; Kagaayi 2005 [S40]	Vogt 2015 [S86]	3
Diarrhea/dysentery	Osendarp 2001 [S61]				el–Rafie 1990 [S31]	Tielsch 2008 [S82]	3
Acute respiratory infection	Datta 1987 [S27]					Tielsch 2008 [S82]	2
Mortality:							
Neonatal mortality rate	Bang 2005 [S13]; Baqui 2009 [S14]; Bhutta 2008 [S20]; Bhandari 2013 [S19]; El Arifeen 2012 [S30]; Fottrell 2013 [S33]; Kumar 2008 [S45]; Lewycka 2013 [S47]; Manandhar 2014 [S50]; Perry 2006 [S64]; Persson 2013 [S66]; Rahman 1982 [S68]; Tielsch 2007 [S81]; Tripathy 2010 [S83]	Azad 2010 [S9]; Colbourn 2013 [S24]; Gill 2014 [S34]; Kirkwood 2013 [S44]; More 2012 [S52]; Sloan 2008 [S76]; Soofi 2012 [S77]	Bang 1999 [S12]; Memon 2015 [S51]; Spencer 1987 [S78]	Singh 2014 [S74]	Rana 2011 [S69]		26

Table 2. *Continued*

OUTCOME MEASURE	ASSESSMENT METHODOLOGY WITH FINDINGS						TOTAL
	Randomized controlled assessments		Non-randomized controlled assessments		Observational (mostly pre/post intervention) assessments		
	Positive effect (n=31)	No significant or negative effect (n=12)	Positive effect (n=8)	No significant or negative effect (n=2)	Positive effect (n=13)	No significant or negative effect (n=7)	
Early neonatal mortality rate			Memon 2015 [S51]	Singh 2014 [S74]			2
Perinatal mortality rate	Bang 2005 [S13]; Bhutta 2008 [S20]; Kumar 2008 [S45]; Jokhio 2005 [S39]		Bang 1999 [S12]; Memon 2015 [S51]		Seim 2014 [S72]		7
Early infant mortality rate			Christian 2004 [S22]				1
Infant mortality rate	Lewycka 2015 [S47]; Perry 2006 [S64]; Shankar 2008 [S73]	Benn 2008 [S18]; Sloan 2008 [S76]	Perry 2006 [S64]		Anand 2000 [S5]; Li 2007 [S48]; ASHA–India 2008 [S7]	Becker 1993 [S17]	9
Sepsis–specific case fatality rate					Khanal 2011 [S42]		1
Diarrhea–specific mortality						el–Rafie 1990 [S31]	1
Tetanus–specific mortality rate		Newell 1996 [S59]			Becker 1993 [S17]; ASHA–India 2008 [S7]; Anand 2000 [S5]		5
Pneumonia–specific mortality rate					Bang 1994 [S11]		1
Low birth weight–specific mortality rate	Sloan 2008 [S76]; Tielsch 2007 [S81]						2
Total number of assessments	31	12	8	2	13	7	73

*See Appendix S2 in **Online Supplementary Document**.

Overall, 31 of the 43 measurements of outcomes of randomized controlled assessments that are shown in Table 2 demonstrated positive effects: 2 out of 4 for nutritional status, 6 out of 6 for morbidity, and 24 out of 34 for mortality. Among the 10 measurements among non–randomized controlled assessments (all of which were mortality assessments), 8 out 10 demonstrated positive effects. Among the uncontrolled observational (mostly pre/post intervention) assessments, 13 out of 20 (65%) demonstrated positive effects.

This analysis indicates that, for a range of indicators, between 65–90% of the assessments included in our analysis observed a positive outcome or a favorable health impact. Among the 43 randomized controlled trials (RCTs), 31 (72%) showed a positive outcome and 12 (28%) showed either no effect or (in one case) a negative effect.

Of the 50 non–randomized and observational assessments included in our analysis (mostly pre/post intervention assessments), 13 out of 20 (65%) demonstrated a positive outcome. Similarly, for the health process/output measures shown in **Table 3**, the findings are strongly favorable. 37 out of 42 (88%) measurements among randomized assessments demonstrative positive effects, as did 28 out of 34 (82%) measurements among non–randomized controlled assessments and 31 out of 36 (86%) measurements among observational studies (which were mostly pre/post intervention assessments).

Table S1 in **Online Supplementary Document** provides details of the 43 randomized controlled trials included among our assessments.

Implementation strategies

A more detailed analysis of community–based implementation strategies for improving maternal, neonatal and child health is contained in another article in this series [12]. However, here we mention some of the findings that relate specifically to neonatal health interventions.

Key intervention implementation strategies that were utilized in CBPHC projects that improved neonatal health included: home visitation by CHWs for education in relation to prevention, recognition of danger signs, and early treatment/referral of neonates with serious illnesses; community–based treatment and early referral by CHWs for neonatal sepsis; outreach from health facilities, especially for antenatal care and maternal immunization against neonatal tetanus; and participatory women's groups (sometimes referred to as support groups) to raise awareness about healthy practices during pregnancy and for the newborn, and to raise awareness of danger signs for which facility–based care should be sought.

Table 3. *Assessments of community–based primary health care projects that document improvements in neonatal health as defined by health process/output indicators**

PROCESS AND OUTPUT MEASURES	ASSESSMENT METHODOLOGY WITH FINDINGS						TOTAL
	Randomized controlled assessments		Non-randomized controlled assessments		Observational (mostly pre/post intervention) assessments		
	Positive effect (n = 36)	No useful or negative effect (n = 5)	Positive effect (n = 28)	No useful or negative effect (n = 5)	Positive effect (n = 31)	No useful or negative effect (n = 5)	
Newborn care practices:							
Thermal care	Kumar 2008 [S45]; Findley 2013 [S32]	Sloan 2008 [S76]	Khan 2013 [S41]; Syed 2006 [S79]				5
Colostrum administration	Kumar 2008 [S45]		Khan 2013 [S41]; Memon 2015 [S51]	Malekafzali 2000 [S49]	Vir 2013 [S85]		5
Cord cleansing with chlorhexidine	El Arifeen 2012 [S30]; Mullany 2006 [S53]; Mullany 2013 [S54]; Soofi 2012 [S77]				Orabaton 2015 [S60]		5
Delayed bathing of the newborn within the first six hours after birth	Kumar 2008 [S45]; Penfold 2014 [S63]		Khan 2013 [S41]		Sitrin 2015 [S75]		4
Clean hygiene practices for home delivery	Fottrell 2013 [S33]; Kumar 2008 [S45]; Penfold 2014 [S63]		Memon 2015 [S51]; Khan 2013 [S41]		Parashar 2013 [S62]; Sitrin 2015 [S75]		7
Knowledge on newborn health:							
Knowledge of newborn danger signs	Findley 2013 [S32]		Khan 2013 [S41]		Callaghan–Koru 2013 [S21]; Dongre 2009 [S29]		4
Knowledge on early breastfeeding			Malekafzali 2000 [S49]				1
Knowledge on feeding during diarrhea episodes			Malekafzali 2000 [S49]				1
Feeding practices and micronutrient supplementation:							

Table 3. Continued

PROCESS AND OUTPUT MEASURES	ASSESSMENT METHODOLOGY WITH FINDINGS						TOTAL
	Randomized controlled assessments		Non-randomized controlled assessments		Observational (mostly pre/post intervention) assessments		
	Positive effect (n = 36)	No useful or negative effect (n = 5)	Positive effect (n = 28)	No useful or negative effect (n = 5)	Positive effect (n = 31)	No useful or negative effect (n = 5)	
Breastfeeding within the first two hours	Findley 2013 [S32]		Memon 2015 [S51]; Crookston 2000 [S26]; Syed 2006 [S79]	Malekafzali 2000 [S49]	Vir 2013 [S85]	Khan 2013 [S41]	7
Proper feeding during diarrhea episodes				Malekafzali 2000 [S49]			1
Exclusive breastfeeding	Bashour 2008 [S16]; Coutinho 2005 [S25]; Haider 2000 [S37]; Qureshi 2011 [S67]; Rotheram-Borus 2014 [S71]; Kimani-Murage 2015 [S43]; Lewycka 2013 [S47]		Balaluka 2012 [S10]; Crookston 2000 [S26]; Haider 2002 [S38]; Khan 2013 [S41]	Malekafzali 2000 [S49]	Neumann 1993 [S57]; Thiam 1995 [S80]	Khan 2013 [S41]; Neumann 1999 [S57]; Neutzling 1993 [S58]	17
Micronutrient supplementation coverage	Bang 2005 [S13]; Benn 2008 [S18]; Daulaire 1992 [S28]; Osendarp 2001 [S61]; Shankar 2008 [S73]	Christian 2003 [S23]				Tielsch 2008 [S82]	7
Referral and treatment of health conditions:							
Receipt of Amoxicillin within 24 h of onset of pneumonia symptoms					Murray 2014 [S55]		1
Referral of sick newborns	Ansah Manu 2014 [S6]	Bhutta 2008 [S20]	Baqui 2008 [S15]				3
Treatment of diarrhea with ORT					Thiam 1995 [S80]		1
Accuracy of assessments and adherence to protocols:							

Table 3. *Continued*

PROCESS AND OUTPUT MEASURES	ASSESSMENT METHODOLOGY WITH FINDINGS						TOTAL
	Randomized controlled assessments		Non–randomized controlled assessments		Observational (mostly pre/post intervention) assessments		
	Positive effect (n = 36)	No useful or negative effect (n = 5)	Positive effect (n = 28)	No useful or negative effect (n = 5)	Positive effect (n = 31)	No useful or negative effect (n = 5)	
Correct determination of low birth weight and very low birth weight by CHWs					Amano 2015 [S4]		1
Error free management of cases of pneumonia by traditional birth attendants			Perry 2016 [S65]				1
Correct interpretation of growth chart by mothers			Malekafzali 2000 [S49]				1
Detection/identification of sick newborns	Ansah Manu 2014 [S6]		Baqui 2008 [S15]		Rana 2011 [S69]		3
Adherence to protocols for management of LBW and VLBW					Amano 2015 [S4]		1
Health care utilization and birth preparedness:							
Antenatal care attendance	Persson 2013 [S66]		Uzondu 2015 [S84]; Baqui 2008 [S15]	Memon 2015 [S51]	Wangalwa 2012 [S88]; AFK–Pakistan 2014 [S1]; Rana 2011 [S69]		7
Delivery in a health facility or by a skilled birth attendant	Bhutta 2008 [S20]; Colbourn 2013 [S24]		Memon 2015 [S51]; Uzondu 2015 [S84]; Khan 2013 [S41]		AFK–Pakistan 2014 [S1]; Awoonor–Williams 2004 [S8]; Gopinath 2011 [S35]; Murray 2014 [S55]; Wangalwa 2012 [S88]		10

Table 3. *Continued*

Process and output measures	Assessment methodology with findings						Total
	Randomized controlled assessments		Non-randomized controlled assessments		Observational (mostly pre/post intervention) assessments		
	Positive effect (n = 36)	No useful or negative effect (n = 5)	Positive effect (n = 28)	No useful or negative effect (n = 5)	Positive effect (n = 31)	No useful or negative effect (n = 5)	
Receipt of postnatal care	Findley 2013 [S32]	Bashour 2008 [S16]			AFK–Pakistan 2014 [S1]; Wangalwa 2012 [S88]		4
Care seeking for neonatal illnesses	Bhandari 2013 [S19]; Ansah Manu 2014 [S6]			Ali 2005 [S3]	Murray 2014 [S55]; Nalwadda 2013 [S56]; Dongre 2009 [S29]		6
Immunization coverage	Rahman 1982 [S68]; Findley 2013 [S32]	Bashour 2008 [S16]	Memon 2015 [S51]		Becker 1993 [S17]; Nalwadda 2013 [S56]		6
Participation in group activities					Gopinath 2011 [S35]		1
Birth preparedness	Waiswa 2015 [S87]		Perry 2016 [S65]				2
Total number of assessments	37	5	28	6	31	5	111

ORT – oral rehydration therapy, LBW – low birth weight, VLBW – very low birth weight

*See Appendix S2 in **Online Supplementary Document.**

As shown in **Figure 3**, the most common associated implementation strategies were the training of CHWs (carried out in 75% of the projects) and the formation of women's support groups (present in 36% of the projects).

As shown in **Figure 4**, over half of the projects had stated goals and associated activities of promoting women's or community empowerment, forging links between the community and the health system and promoting local resource use. Less–commonly stated goals and activities were promotion of community leadership, adaptive learning and promotion of equity.

The data extraction form asked reviewers to subjectively judge whether the assessment observed any effect of community participation on health outcome and whether or not the outcome was positive. In 65% (60) of the 93 reports, community participation was reported to have had an effect, and in all of these cases the effect was judged to be positive. In over half (52%) of the 93 reports, the reviewers judged that the linkages between the community and the health system had an impact on health outcomes, and the effect on neonatal health was positive in almost all (93%) of these cases.

Equity

In terms of coverage, community–based efforts are generally designed to be more equitable than facility–based approaches in reaching those most in need and in improving the health of the most disadvantaged. This arises from the

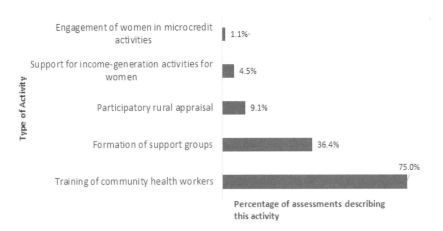

Figure 3. *Common associated activities carried out in the implementation of CBPHC projects to improve neonatal health (n = 93). The sum is greater than 100% since some projects had more than one of these activities.*

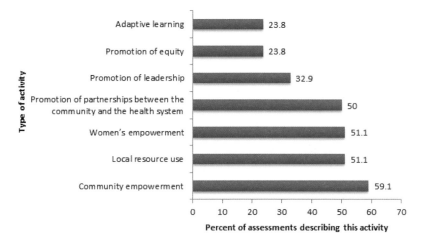

Figure 4. *Common associated goals and activities carried out in the implementation of CBPHC projects to improve neonatal health (n = 93). The sum is greater than 100% since many projects employed more than one strategy.*

fact that community–based approaches contain strong outreach elements and are often able to reach those who have difficulties in accessing facility–based health care, whether because of distance or socioeconomic challenges such as cost or other barriers. The equity effects assessed among all the child health projects in our database are described elsewhere [13]. Here, however, we present the findings specific to neonatal health projects.

In total, 8 of the 93 assessments in our neonatal health review examined equity of health outcomes, using different categories of equity (income, geography, etc.). Of the 10 equity assessments reported for these 10 projects, 7 (70%) were considered to be "pro–equitable" (ie, the outcomes were <u>more</u> favorable for the newborns in the most disadvantaged households). For one equity assessment (10%), the outcome was considered to be "equitable" (ie, the outcome was equally favorable in the most disadvantaged and other households), and in only two equity assessment (20%) the outcomes were "inequitable" (ie, the outcomes were less favorable for newborns in the most disadvantaged households compared to other households) (**Figure 4**).

DISCUSSION

Our analysis provides strong evidence that CBPHC can improve neonatal health in low–income settings. Of the studies with strong experimental research designs, over 70% showed a positive neonatal health impact. Although

Table 4. *Equity assessments of community–based primary health care in improving neonatal health**

OUTCOME OF ASSESSMENT	OUTCOME INDICATOR	EQUITY CATEGORY	REFERENCE
Pro–equitable	**Mortality**		
	Neonatal mortality rate	Geography	ASHA–India 2008 [S7])
	Neonatal mortality rate	Geography	Bang 1999 [S12]
	Perinatal mortality rate	Geography	Bang 2005 [S13], Bang 1999 [S12]
	Postnatal care		
	Postnatal care coverage	Socio–economic status (including education)	Awoonor–Williams 2004 [S8]
	Skilled birth attendance		
	Skilled attendant at birth	Socio–economic status (including education)	Awoonor–Williams 2004 [S8]
	Breastfeeding		
	Exclusive breastfeeding from birth to 6 mo	Geography	Crookston 2000 [S26]
	Breastfeeding initiation within the first hour of life	Geography	Crookston 2000 [S26]
Equitable	**Mortality**		
	Tetanus neonatorum mortality rate	Geography	Newell 1966 [S59]
Inequitable	**Mortality**		
	Neonatal morality rate	Socio–economic status	Razzaque 2007 [S70]
	Breastfeeding		
	Exclusive breastfeeding from birth to 6 mo	Socio–economic status	Coutinho 2005 [S25]

*See Appendix S2 in **Online Supplementary Document**.

many of these studies were smaller scale pilots or efficacy studies, it demonstrates that CBPHC can be an essential tool where access to facilities is limited and many births take place at home. In these settings, access to antenatal care is often limited; for example, only 49% of pregnant women in sub–Saharan Africa obtain four antenatal care visits [1]. Furthermore, among the 75 countries with the greatest burden of neonatal mortality, the median national coverage of interventions that are important for improving neonatal mortality is quite low: 65% for skilled attendant at delivery, 28% for postnatal visits for newborns, and 50% for early initiation of breastfeeding [14]. Community–based approaches will be essential for the near term in order to achieve universal coverage of health services for these mothers during their delivery and immediately following birth. Even if primary health care services are better developed and facility coverage of antenatal, delivery, and postnatal care increases, CBPHC can continue to make a contribution to improved neonatal health through promotion of healthy household practices and awareness of danger signs for which facility–based care should be sought.

The most common outcome indicators used in the assessments included in our analysis were related to population coverage of postnatal care and exclusive breastfeeding during the neonatal period; mortality was also relatively well–studied. While our review did not include assessments of the quality of implemented interventions or the degree to which projects were implemented under ideal vs more routine conditions (to assess to what degree the assessments were of CBPHC efficacy as opposed to effectiveness), we did summarize the findings by the rigor of the study design and demonstrated that for all levels of methodological rigor, CBPHC approaches appeared to produce favorable outcomes on neonatal health. It is worth noting the importance of assessing and improving the quality of care provided at the time of health contacts between patients and providers, whether they take place in facilities or in homes; however, information on this topic was missing in almost all of the assessments included in our analysis. Further, many of the studies with the strongest designs also had the most intensive support in carrying out the intervention, making it more difficult to judge the effectiveness if scaled up without focused attention or resources.

Our analysis reveals that many of the leading causes of death among children during the first month of life – especially those caused by infection – can be effectively addressed at the community level by CHWs if they have proper training and support. Home–based neonatal care includes promotion of immediate and exclusive breastfeeding, promotion of cleanliness, application of a topical antiseptic (chlorhexidine) to the umbilical cord, prevention of hypothermia, and early diagnosis and referral for treatment of neonatal sepsis. Strong evidence was found for the capacity of CHWs to promote clean delivery, especially in settings where births occur at home and hygiene is poor, to improve neonatal care practices at home, and to identify sick neonates in need of further care and treatment for certain conditions.

Given that many neonatal care projects utilize community health workers (CHWs), it is expected that many interventions can be provided close to or in the home, especially if CHWs live near their patients. Key community–based intervention strategies that were demonstrated to be successful in our analysis include home visitation by CHWs to educate mothers about healthy household practices, danger signs, the importance of early referral and treatment of neonates with danger signs, and outreach by mobile teams from health facilities (especially to provide maternal immunization against neonatal tetanus). Additionally, our analysis identifies the capacity of participatory women's groups to raise awareness about healthy practices during pregnancy and the postpartum/postnatal period, and to educate about danger signs for which facility–based care should be sought and the favorable effects of this approach for reducing neonatal mortality. Our equity analysis shows that almost all of the CBPHC interventions for improving newborn health benefit more disadvantaged groups to a greater degree than others.

This study had a number of limitations. The evidence is derived from projects mostly in rural South Asia. Most projects had a relatively short timeline and so we are unable to ascertain if they were successful in the long term. Furthermore, many (but not all) of the projects were implemented in relatively small populations under relatively ideal circumstances in which high–quality training, supervision, and logistical support were assured. So whether similar results can be achieved under more routine condition in larger populations over long periods of time is not known at present.

The large proportion of positive outcomes could be partially due to publication bias. Especially given that all study types were included (such as gray literature reports), there may have been a tendency by organizations to promote their successful work and only publish studies which had a beneficial impact. This study was further limited by the wide range of definitions, indicators and measurements used, which made standardization impossible. We aimed to provide useful categories and definitions, but the variation is wide. For example, it is known that the capacity and competence of CHWs varies widely; further analysis of the details regarding how CHWs were trained and deployed in the projects included in our review were limited. The context in which projects were carried out is also wide: details regarding exactly how the intervention strategies were carried out, and the specific conditions required for them to be effective at scale, go beyond the scope of this analysis. Finally, while this is intended to be a comprehensive review, the field is vast and some studies may not have been included.

The need to accelerate declines in neonatal mortality is readily apparent. In order to achieve universal health coverage and to end preventable neonatal deaths by the year 2030, basic and essential evidence–based neonatal health care interventions will need to reach all mothers and their newborns. Since many countries will not be able to provide universal coverage of essential newborn services by 2030 through facility–based services, progress in reducing neonatal mortality in high–mortality, resource–constrained settings will have to partially depend for the foreseeable future upon strengthening the types of interventions and approaches described here, and on improving timely referral to facilities for newborns with complications. The next step in this process is to test the types of interventions and approaches described here at scale using rigorous operations research methodologies. Further research is also needed in a wider variety of geographic areas, in urban and peri–urban settings, and for longer–term programs.

According to one recently published analysis based on modeling tools [2], immediately scaling up the currently available community–based interventions with evidence of effectiveness for reducing neonatal mortality to reach 90% population coverage would avert an estimated 740 000 neonatal deaths annually (27.4% of the total of 2.7 million neonatal deaths currently occurring each year). Similarly, a separate analysis [15] estimates that 700 000 newborn lives that would be saved if all of the community–based interventions gradually achieved a coverage of 90% over a 5–year period. While CBPHC approaches for reducing the number of stillbirths were not included in this review, there is growing evidence that community–based efforts to improve antenatal care, especially nutrition and malaria prevention, will have effects on the prevalence of stillbirth worldwide [15]. If the interventions that can be provided at primary health care centers and at hospitals but not in the community (eg, full supportive care for preterm newborns or treatment if very serious infection) were able to reach 90% of the neonates who need them, an additional 760 00 neonatal deaths could be averted (170 000 at primary health care centers and 0.59 million at hospitals) [2]. Thus, even though facility–based care is important for improving neonatal health, expanding the coverage of community–based services will also be essential in order to quickly accelerate the decline of neonatal mortality in high–burden countries.

CONCLUSIONS

The evidence regarding the potential of CBPHC to improve neonatal health in resource–constrained settings is strong. Now there is a need to begin to assemble evidence regarding the effectiveness of implementation of these interventions and strategies at scale. The scaling up of effective community–based interventions will be essential for accelerating progress in reducing neonatal mortality in the near term and for reaching universal coverage of evidence–based interventions for improving neonatal health. Based upon the current evidence, this will require the development and strengthening of a community–based platform involving (1) training and deployment of CHWs to visit homes frequently to promote healthy household behaviors, identification of neonates in need of referral, and utilization of health facilities appropriately, (2) formation and support of participatory women's groups, and (3) strengthening of outreach services provided by mobile health teams for provision of antenatal and postnatal care. Identifying ways for all newborns to receive the highest quality of care that can be provided in the home will have a sizable impact on neonatal mortality and morbidity worldwide.

Acknowledgements: The authors wish to thank Steve Hodgins, Abhay Bang and Zulfi Bhutta for comments on earlier drafts of this manuscript, and the many students and research assistants who contributed to the assembling the database and the analysis. We are grateful to the following organizations that provided small grants to cover the expenses of this review: UNICEF, the World Bank, the Department of Child and Adolescent Health and Development of the World Health Organization, the CORE Group (Collaboration and Resources for Child Health)/USAID, Future Generations, and the Gates Foundation. We are also grateful to the American Public Health Association and particularly its International Health Section staff, which administered some of these funds. We thank Future Generations for providing office space, administrative support, and salary support to Dr Perry during the initial phase of the review. The World Bank made it possible for one of its consultants, Dr Bahie Rassekh, to participate as a member of the Study Team.

Funding: The following organizations provided funds that were used to conduct the work described in this article: The World Health Organization, UNICEF, the World Bank, the United States Agency for International Development, and the Gates Foundation. The organizations that provided financial support had no role in the execution of the review.

Authorship declaration: ES wrote the first draft. ES, KS and PF conducted the primary analysis of the data. All of the authors participated in the revision of earlier drafts and approved the final draft.

Conflict of interest: All authors have completed the Unified Competing Interest Form at www.icmje.org/coi_disclosure.pdf (available upon request from the corresponding author), and declare no conflict of interest.

References

1   UNICEF. The State of the World's Children 2016: A Fair Chance for Every Child. 2016. Available: http://www.unicef.org/sowc2016/. Accessed: 25 April 2017.

2   Black RE, Levin C, Walker N, Chou D, Liu L, Temmerman M, et al. Reproductive, maternal, newborn, and child health: key messages from Disease Control Priorities 3rd Edition. Lancet. 2016;388:2811-24.

3   Oza S, Cousens SN, Lawn JE. Estimation of daily risk of neonatal death, including the day of birth, in 186 countries in 2013: a vital-registration and modelling-based study. Lancet Glob Health. 2014;2:e635-44. Medline:25442688 doi:10.1016/S2214-109X(14)70309-2

4   Baqui AH, Mitra D, Begum N, Hurt L, Soremekun S, Edmond K, et al. Neonatal mortality within 24 hours of birth in six low- and lower-middle-income countries. Bull World Health Organ. 2016;94:752-58B. Medline:27843165 doi:10.2471/BLT.15.160945

5   Liu L, Johnson HL, Cousens S, Perin J, Scott S, Lawn JE, et al. Global, regional, and national causes of child mortality: an updated systematic analysis for 2010 with time trends since 2000. Lancet. 2012;379:2151-61. Medline:22579125 doi:10.1016/S0140-6736(12)60560-1

6   Black R, Laxminarayan R, Temmerman M, Walker N, editors. Disease Control Priorities: Reproductive, Maternal, Newborn, and Child Health, Third Edition. Washington, DC: World Bank; 2016.

7   Lassi ZS, Kumar R, Bhutta ZA. Community-based care to improve maternal, newborn, and child health. 2016. In: Disease Control Priorities: Reproductive, Maternal, Newborn, and Child Health. Washington, DC: World Bank. Available: https://openknowledge.worldbank.org/bitstream/handle/10986/23833/9781464803482.pdf?sequence=3&isAllowed=y. Accessed: 26 April 2017.

8   Bhutta ZA, Darmstadt GL, Hasan BS, Haws RA. Community-based interventions for improving perinatal and neonatal health outcomes in developing countries: a review of the evidence. Pediatrics. 2005;115:519-617. Medline:15866863 doi:10.1542/peds.2004-1441

9   Gogia S, Sachdev HP. Home-based neonatal care by community health workers for preventing mortality in neonates in low- and middle-income countries: a systematic review. J Perinatol. 2016;36 Suppl 1:S55-73. Medline:27109093 doi:10.1038/jp.2016.33

10 Perry H, Rassekh B, Gupta S, Wilhelm J, Freeman P. Comprehensive review of the evidence regarding the effectiveness of community-based primary health care in improving maternal, neonatal and child health: 1. rationale, methods and database description. J Glob Health. 2017;7:010901.

11 Donabedian A. The quality of care. How can it be assessed? JAMA. 1988;260:1743-8. Medline:3045356 doi:10.1001/jama.1988.03410120089033

12 Perry HB, Sacks E, Schleiff M, Kumapley R, Gupta S. Comprehensive review of the evidence regarding the effectiveness of community-based primary health care in improving maternal, neonatal and child health: 6. strategies used by effective projects. J Glob Health. 2017;7:010906.

13 Schleiff M, Kumapley R, Freeman P, Gupta S, Rassekh B, Perry HB. Comprehensive review of the evidence regarding the effectiveness of community-based primary health care in improving maternal, neonatal and child health: 5. equity effects. J Glob Health. 2017;7:010905.

14 Victora CG, Requejo JH, Barros AJ, Berman P, Bhutta Z, Boerma T, et al. Countdown to 2015: a decade of tracking progress for maternal, newborn, and child survival. Lancet. 2016;387:2049-59. Medline:26477328 doi:10.1016/S0140-6736(15)00519-X

15 Chou VB, Friberg I, Christian M, Walker N, Perry HB. How many lives of mothers and children could be averted by strengthening community-based primary health care? An analysis using the lives saved (LiST) tool. J Glob Health. 2017;2:020401.

Acknowledgement: originally published as: Emma Sacks, Paul A Freeman, Kwame Sakyi, Mary Carol Jennings, Bahie M Rassekh, Sundeep Gupta, Henry B Perry:Comprehensive review of the evidence regarding the effectiveness of Community–Based Primary Health Care in improving maternal, neonatal and child health:3. neonatal health findings. Reprinted with permission from Edinburgh University Global Health Society under Creative Commons Attribution Licence (Journal of Global Health 2017; 010903).

Comprehensive review of the evidence regarding the effectiveness of community–based primary health care in improving maternal, neonatal and child health: 4. child health findings

Paul A Freeman[1,2], Meike Schleiff[3], Emma Sacks[3], Bahie M Rassekh[4], Sundeep Gupta[5], Henry B Perry[3]

[1] Independent consultant, Seattle, Washington, USA
[2] University of Washington School of Public Health, Seattle, Washington, USA
[3] Department of International Health, Johns Hopkins Bloomberg School of Public Health, Baltimore, Maryland, USA
[4] The World Bank, Washington, District of Columbia, USA
[5] Medical Epidemiologist, Lusaka, Zambia

Background This paper assesses the effectiveness of community–based primary health care (CBPHC) in improving child health beyond the neonatal period. Although there has been an accelerated decline in global under–5 mortality since 2000, mortality rates remain high in much of sub–Saharan Africa and in some south Asian countries where under–5 mortality is also decreasing more slowly. Essential interventions for child health at the community level have been identified. Our review aims to contribute further to this knowledge by examining how strong the evidence is and exploring in greater detail what specific interventions and implementation strategies appear to be effective.

Methods We reviewed relevant documents from 1950 onwards using a detailed protocol. Peer reviewed documents, reports and books assessing the impact of one or more CBPHC interventions on child health (defined as changes in population coverage of one or more key child survival interventions, nutritional status, serious morbidity or mortality) among children in a geographically defined population were examined for inclusion. Two separate reviews took place of each document followed by an independent consolidated summative review. Data from the latter review were transferred to an electronic database for analysis.

Results The findings provide strong evidence that the major causes of child mortality in resource–constrained settings can be addressed at the community level largely by engaging communities and supporting community–level workers. For all major categories of interventions (nutritional interventions; control of pneumonia, diarrheal disease and malaria; HIV prevention and treatment; immunizations; integrated management of childhood diseases; and comprehensive primary health care) we have presented randomized controlled trials that have consistently produced statistically significant and operationally important effects.

Conclusions This review shows that there is strong evidence of effectiveness for CBPHC implementation of an extensive range of interventions to improve child health and that four major strategies for delivering these interventions are effective.

This paper concentrates on the effectiveness of community–based primary health care (CBPHC) in improving the health of children beyond the neonatal period. In 2015, the global mortality rate for children younger than 5 years of age (referred to hereafter as under–5 mortality) was 42.5 per 1000 live births, a decline from 90.4 per 1000 live births in 1990 [1]. Although there has been an accelerated decline in global under–5 mortality since 2000, mortality rates remain high in much of sub–Saharan Africa and in some south Asian countries where under–5 mortality is also decreasing more slowly [1]. Following the neonatal period (when 45% of under–5 deaths occur currently), the major causes of mortality in children are pneumonia (26% of deaths in this age group), diarrhea (18%), and malaria (12%) [2]. Undernutrition is a cause of 45% of all under–5 deaths [3].

Essential interventions for child health at the community level have been identified as: promotion of breastfeeding and complementary feeding, supplementation with vitamin A and zinc, immunizations, co–trimoxazole for HIV–positive children, education on the safe disposal of feces and hand washing, distribution and promotion of insecticide–treated bed nets (ITNs) or indoor residual spraying (IRS) or both; detection and treatment or referral of children with severe acute undernutrition; and detection and treatment of pneumonia, malaria and diarrhea without danger signs and referral if danger signs appear [4]. It has been estimated that scaling up these interventions with an essential package of community–based interventions would avert 1.5 million deaths of children 1–59 months each year [1].

Our review aims to contribute further to this knowledge by examining how strong is the evidence for community–based primary health care (CBPHC) and exploring in greater detail what specific activities appear to be effective. Our concern is not just to strengthen the evidence about which interventions work at the community level but who does them and how, what conditions facilitate effectiveness, and what kinds of community–based approaches appear to be most effective. What characteristics do effective CBPHC activities share, and how strong is the evidence that partnerships between communities and health systems are required in order to improve child and maternal health?

The purpose of this paper is to summarize the evidence regarding the effectiveness of CBPHC for improving child health beyond the neonatal period.

METHODS

Our review aims to provide a comprehensive review of documents from 1950 onwards assessing the effectiveness of projects, programs and research studies (hereafter referred to as projects) using a detailed protocol. We examined peer–reviewed articles, reports and books assessing the impact of one or more CBPHC interventions on child health (coverage of a key evidence–based child survival indicator, nutritional status, serious morbidity, or mortality), among children in a geographically defined population. Two independent reviews were carried out and followed by an independent consolidated summative review. Data from the latter review were transferred to an electronic database for analysis. Data analysis took place using EPI INFO version 3.5.4 (Epi Info, US Centers for Disease Control and Prevention, Atlanta, Georgia, USA).

Only those assessments which had clear documentation of the intervention(s) and their impact on child health where included. Outcome measures included were changes in the population coverage of one or more evidence–based interventions; change in nutritional status (as measured by anthropometry, anemia, or assessment of micro–nutrient deficiency); change in the incidence or in the outcome of serious, life–threatening morbidity (such as pneumonia, diarrhea, malaria, and low–birth weight); and change in mortality (infant, 1–4 year, and under–5 mortality). Further details regarding the methodology are reported elsewhere in this series [5].

RESULTS

General findings

There were 548 assessments included in our database for neonates and 1–59 month–old children. The age of the study population was clearly documented as less than one month in 48 of these assessments. In another 12 assessments the intervention was found to focus on neonatal and maternal health. An analysis of these assessments is reported in the other papers in this series focusing on maternal and neonatal health and not reported here [6,7]. The remaining 489 assessments (**Figure 1**) focused predominately on children beyond the neonatal period, but many also include neonates. The complete bibliography of these assessments in contained in Appendix S1 in **Online Supplementary Document,** and are indicated in parenthesis with a prefix S throughout this paper.

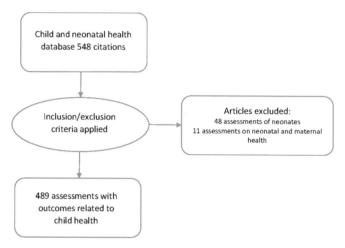

Figure 1. *Flowchart of selection of assessments for child health review.*

Table 1 below lists the most common child interventions described in these 489 assessments. All but 5 of the 129 projects that were classified as providing "primary health care" also implemented one or more of the other interventions shown in **Table 1**. Some categories of child interventions had a relatively small number of assessments and so have been grouped as Other Interventions in **Table 1**. These Other interventions are not analyzed in detail in this paper. Other intervention categories not included above and included in the "Others" group in **Table 1** focused on trachoma prevention, tuberculosis, community organizations, financing, training and use of radios.

Table 2 shows the frequency of assessments according to the number of interventions implemented (not including "primary health care" and counting Integrated Management of Childhood Illness as one intervention). Although half (52%) of the assessments described projects with only one intervention and another quarter (21%) contained only two, one quarter contained three or more.

Below we provide an analysis of the interventions for children beyond the neonatal period grouped according to the categories listed in **Table 1**. The full list of studies reviewed and referred to in the parentheses in the text below can be found in Appendix S2 in **Online Supplementary Document**, where the assessments in our review that are cited here can be identified from the number in brackets in the text.

Table 3 outlines the types of study methodologies used for these 489 studies. One–half (52%) are controlled studies and one–quarter (26%) are uncontrolled, before–after comparisons. Other types of study methodologies make up the other quarter of assessments. These various study methodologies are spread

Table 1. *Leading categories of child health interventions included in assessments*

INTERVENTION AREA	No.*	PERCENTAGE (N = 489)
Any nutrition–related activity (growth monitoring, breastfeeding promotion, complementary feeding promotion, or provision of micronutrients)	255	52.2
Diarrhea prevention or treatment	183	37.4
Diarrhea prevention and treatment	98	20.0
Diarrhea prevention only	48	9.8
Diarrhea treatment only	30	6.1
Malaria prevention or treatment	150	30.3
Malaria prevention and treatment	91	18.6
Malaria prevention only	27	5.5
Malaria treatment only	11	2.2
Immunizations	132	27.0
Primary health care	129	26.4
Integrated Management of Childhood Illness	110	22.5
Pneumonia prevention or treatment	108	22.1
Pneumonia prevention and treatment	46	9.4
Pneumonia prevention only	19	3.9
Pneumonia treatment only	40	8.2
HIV prevention or HIV/AIDS treatment	42	8.6
HIV prevention and HIV/AIDS treatment	13	2.7
HIV prevention only	24	4.9
HIV/AIDS treatment only	2	0.0
Other	24	4.9

*The sum of this column exceeds 489 since many assessments described more than one intervention.

Table 2. *Number of intervention category areas among projects that focused on children beyond the neonatal period*

NUMBER OF INTERVENTIONS PER PROJECT	FREQUENCY	PERCENTAGE (%)
1	243	51.6
2	97	21.3
3 to 4	76	16.6
5 to 7	49	10.5
Projects with interventions categorized as "Other"	24	4.9
Total	489	100.0

Table 3. *Type of study methodology used among child health assessments*

TYPE OF STUDY	FREQUENCY	PERCENTAGE (%)
Randomized, controlled	177	36.6
Non–randomized, controlled	74	15.3
Uncontrolled, before–after	127	26.3
Case–control, cross–sectional	15	3.1
Cross–sectional	45	9.3
Descriptive	27	5.6
Non–study activity	24	4.3
Total	489	100.0

fairly evenly across the major intervention categorical areas listed in **Table 1** (data not shown).

Space limitations prevent us from a detailed analysis of all 489 assessments (as presented in Appendix S1 in **Online Supplementary Document**). We focus on those assessments that have the strongest study designs and greatest size of significant effects (these are presented in Appendix S2 in Online Supplementary Document). The remaining assessments in our review had similar effects unless otherwise stated.

Findings specific to pneumonia and diarrhea

Pneumonia is the leading single cause of under–5 mortality globally, accounting for 18% of deaths [2]. Diarrhea is a major cause of child mortality and morbidity globally and is responsible for 9% of deaths of children younger than 5 years of age [2]. Under the Integrated Global Action Plan for Pneumonia and Diarrhea (GAPPD), actions to address pneumonia and diarrhea are integrated according to a Treat, Protect and Prevent framework [8]. We will follow this framework in presenting our findings.

Treat

This part of the framework includes diagnosis, screening, triage and treatment. Our review includes five randomized controlled studies (RCTs) that all showed operationally important and statistically significant reductions in child mortality as a result of community health worker (CHW) treatment of pneumonia with antibiotics – reductions in the range of 13% to 60% [S1–5]. Throughout this article we will be referencing assessments from our database with numbers in brackets, preceded by an S prefix, to distinguish them from the references cited in the list of references at the end of this article. The number in brackets with an S prefix refers to the number of the assessment in Appendix S2 in **Online Supplementary Document**. Many other assessments – mainly non–randomized controlled, uncontrolled and case–control studies – also observed significant operationally important decreases in pneumonia–specific mortality in children aged less than 5 years, ranging from 28% to 69% [S6–11]. Two other RCTs demonstrated that CHWs can decrease the clinical severity of pneumonia significantly by treating respiratory infections at the community level through implementing good–quality case management [S12, S13]. Over 20 other studies showed decreases in child pneumonia–specific incidence or mortality but as their pneumonia case management was part of Integrated

Management of Childhood Illnesses (IMCI) or Primary Health Care (PHC), they will be discussed under those sections below. Co–trimoxazole was the antibiotic most commonly used by CHWs in these studies.

Protect

Under this component are good health practices from birth: exclusive breast-feeding during the first six months of life, adequate complementary feeding, and vitamin A supplementation. Several RCTs demonstrated the efficacy of community–based vitamin A supplementation in reducing pneumonia mortality. In one, vitamin A supplementation decreased pneumonia–specific child mortality by 26% [S14]. In another study, the incidence of pneumonia was decreased through vitamin A supplementation by 44% [S15]. Zinc supplementation and promotion of hand washing provided by CHWs were each also found to significantly decrease the incidence of both pneumonia and diarrhea [S16, S17]. In one randomized controlled trial assessment, a community–based integrated nutrition program apparently not including vitamin A or zinc supplementation demonstrated a decreased incidence of pneumonia [S18]. Studies of vitamin A and zinc supplementation will be presented in more detail under the nutrition section below. Further studies have demonstrated the strong efficacy of zinc supplementation in reducing the incidence, severity and/or duration of diarrheal episodes in children [S19–24].

Prevent

This component includes vaccinations, hand washing with soap, safe drinking water and sanitation, reducing household air pollution, HIV prevention and co–trimoxazole prophylaxis for HIV–infected and HIV–exposed children. Education of community members about diarrheal disease was a common activity carried out by trained CHWs, usually by visiting households or meeting with community groups. Randomized controlled trials found that community education focused specifically on the importance of proper disposal of animal feces from living areas produced decreases in the incidence of childhood diarrhea [S25, S26]. Randomized controlled trial assessments of education of caregivers about hand washing along with the provision of soap also decreased childhood diarrhea to an even greater degree than those mentioned in the previous sentence [S27–31]. Teaching mothers to use oral rehydration solution at home along with education about good household sanitation practices – whether by nurses working at the community level or by CHWs – was also effective [S32–34].

Purification of water within the household with sodium hypochlorite or another locally produced purifying agent was found effective in reducing childhood diarrhea in several studies [S35–38]. Solar sterilization of water was demonstrated as an effective approach to decrease the incidence of childhood diarrhea [S39–41]. Water filters such as BioSand and Lifestraw Family Filter that remove particulate matter were similarly effective in reducing the *E. coli* concentration in water and decreasing episodes of diarrhea [S42, S43]. The efficacy of community–based interventions concerning immunizations, HIV and nutrition are presented later in the respective sections.

Findings specific to malaria

Malaria is one of the three commonest causes of child mortality in those countries where it is endemic. In Africa, malaria is the cause of 15% of under–5 mortality [2]. Major community–based interventions for malaria prevention and treatment include: distribution of insecticide–treated bed nets (ITNs), household residual spraying, antimalarial treatment within the patient's household (HH) or in the community by CHWs, and intermittent preventive treatment (IPT) of malaria with anti–malarial medication. Community–based diagnosis of cases of malaria by CHWs may be based on clinical signs only or assisted by a rapid diagnostic test (RDT). **Table 4** presents illustrative randomized controlled trials from our database.

As shown in **Table 4**, there are now a number of randomized controlled trials of community–based interventions for malaria prevention and control that have shown operationally important programmatic effects, with some showing marked mortality impacts. These assessments demonstrate strong evidence of the effectiveness of community–based approaches to the prevention and control of malaria. The interventions presented include use of CHWs involved in house–to–house and group implementation strategies, treatment of malaria within the community by CHWs and mothers, engagement of women's groups, and malaria control provided by mobile teams from peripheral health facilities.

There were several other assessments that provided evidence in support of the community–based distribution of impregnated bed nets for prevention of malaria [S62–68]. A commonly used approach which produced operationally important outcomes was combining the distribution of ITNs with measles vaccination at the time of mobile clinic outreach sessions [S69–72]. Combining distribution of ITNs with malaria treatment was also effective [S73–75]. Several studies provided evidence that impregnated curtains have some effectiveness

Table 4. Randomized controlled trials of community–based malaria prevention and treatment projects focusing on children

Intervention	Type of outcome	Population size of study area	Specific outcome	Effect compared to control	Statistical significance	Reference number*
Distribution of impregnated bed nets with community education:						
Distribution with education	Mortality	5000–10 000 children in each arm	Mortality among children 1–7 y; mortality among children 1 mo–4 y; all–cause (1 to <5 y) mortality	Decreased by 25%; decreased by 18%; decreased by 33%	0.01; 0.05; 0.01	[S44], [S45], [S46]
Distribution with education	Mortality	2260 children 6 mo to <6 y	Malaria–specific mortality among children 1 to <5 y	Decreased by 30%	0.05	[S47]
Distribution with education	Coverage and mortality	Children in 160 villages	Percentage of children 0 to <5y sleeping under an ITN; child mortality	Increased by 72%; decreased by 12%	0.01; 0.05	[S48], [S48]
Distribution with education	Coverage and morbidity	Children in 8 villages	ITN coverage to all households; *A. gambiensis* density	Increased by 99%; decreased by 99%	0.001, 0.001	[S49], [S49]
LLITN given plus training given to head of household	Morbidity	Children in 2015 households	Percentage of children 0 to <5 y with malaria	Decreased by 38%	0.05	[S50]
Distribution without education	Morbidity	219 children in 16 villages	Percentage of patients with fever	Decreased by 72%	<0.001	[S51]
Distribution with education (CHW going house to house)	Coverage	1400 children	Percentage of children sleeping under an ITN	Increased by 27%	0.05	[S52]
Community health network to support LLITN distribution	Coverage	11 villages	Percentage of total population using ITN at time of a 6-month follow up	Increased by 32% (in children 0 to <5 y)	0.001	[S53]
Education via CHW at HH level and community women's groups	Coverage	40 villages	Percentage of total population sleeping under an ITN	Increased by 49%	<0.001	[S54]
Community and household malaria treatment and prophylaxis:						
Treatment with chloroquine by mothers	Mortality	5385 children 0 to <5 y	All-cause child mortality	Decreased by 41%	0.003	[S55]

Table 4. *Continued*

INTERVENTION	TYPE OF OUTCOME	POPULATION SIZE OF STUDY AREA	SPECIFIC OUTCOME	EFFECT COMPARED TO CONTROL	STATISTICAL SIGNIFICANCE	REFERENCE NUMBER*
Training CHWs to treat malaria using an RDT	Accuracy of diagnosis	1457 children 0 to 15 y	Percentage of children treated unnecessarily with ACT	Decreased by 45%	0.001	[S56]
CHW treatment of malaria (based on RDT results), with AL (and also treatment with amoxicillin if symptoms of pneumonia present)	Morbidity	11 400 children 6 mo to <5 y	Percentage of febrile children who received AL; percentage of children diagnosed with pneumonia who received early appropriate treatment	Decreased by 77%; increased by 53%	<0.0001; <0.001	[S57], [S57]
CHW treatment of malaria with ACT (and also treatment with amoxicillin if symptoms of pneumonia present)	Morbidity	609 children 4-59 mo	Percentage of children receiving prompt and appropriate antibiotics	Increased by 34%	<0.001	[S58]
HH treatment of malaria (using an RDT) by CHW plus monthly IPT for 3 mo	Coverage of chemo-prophylaxis; morbidity	500 children 1-10 y (one-half also received IPT)	Incidence of RDT-confirmed malaria in HH + IPT group compared with HH- only group; coverage of children by 3 doses of IPT	Reduced by 85% (compared with HH only group); oncreased by 97%	0.01; 0.001	[S59], [S60]
IPT [Sulfadoxine–pyrimethamine at 3,9, and 15 mo (at time of routine immunization)	Coverage of chemo-prophylaxis	600 children 3 mo of age	Protective efficacy during the intervention period (among children 3–18 mo)	Increased by 22%	<0.0001	[S61]

ACT– Artemisinin combination therapy, AL– Artemether–lumefantrine, BCC– behavior change communication, CHW– Community health worker, IPT– Intermittent preventive treatment, HH– Household, ITN– insecticide–treated bed net, LLIN– Long–lasing insecticide–treated bed net, mo – month(s), RDT– Rapid diagnostic test, WAZ: weight–for–age Z score, WHZ – weight–for–height Z score, y – year(s)
*See Appendix S2 in **Online Supplementary Document**.

in reducing all–cause child mortality [S76, S77]. Some other studies focused on the use of ITNs but did not show as strong evidence individually [S78–83]. Studies which include prevention and treatment of malaria with Integrated Community Case Management of Childhood Illness (IMCI) or with other integrated approaches (such as Care Groups and Primary Health Care) will be presented later in this paper.

The assessments included in **Table 4** above present important aspects of the community–based treatment of malaria. Kidane et al. [S55], by showing that mothers in a remote area of Ethiopia (Tigray) with minimal training could decrease child mortality by diagnosing and treating malaria themselves, illustrated the importance of adapting interventions to local community circumstances as well as the importance of community capacity building. Other studies presented in **Table 4** provide good evidence that CHWs can diagnose and treat malaria in the community in association with the initial management of pneumonia in the same child at the same time [S57, S58]. Several other studies also demonstrated effective treatment of malaria by CHWs in the community alone or in combination with the treatment of concurrent diarrhea or pneumonia [S84–92].

While many of these studies of malaria treatment demonstrated a reduction in malaria–related morbidity or an improvement in CHW performance outcomes related to malaria, some demonstrated important decreases in overall child mortality as well [S93,94]. The cost-effectiveness of combining malaria and pneumonia treatment was studied. However, the findings were inconclusive [S95]. The demonstration of the capacity of CHWs to accurately diagnose malaria using RDTs is also an important finding [S56].

Table 4 also demonstrates the operational effectiveness of community–level IPT provided by CHWs [S59–61]. Several studies have demonstrated evidence of the important role that other members of the community can play in malaria prevention. School teachers, for instance, can provide IPT with a demonstrable impact on child mortality [S96]. However, the assessment reporting this result, although reporting significant operationally important outcomes, did not provide an adequate description of the intervention and therefore the finding needs to be interpreted with caution.

Trained traditional healers and drug vendors can effectively educate mothers about malaria prevention and early treatment [S97, 98]. Some other studies that focused on malaria treatment or IPT at the community level had results that were consistent with our findings above but the strength of evidence was not as strong [S99–111].

Findings specific to human immunodeficiency virus infection

There were fewer studies specifically on HIV/AIDS prevention and control at the community level. One study demonstrated that community–level treatment with co–trimoxazole of HIV–infected adults led to a reduction of 77% in the mortality of their originally HIV–negative, under–10 year–old household members. The provision of the drug and the monitoring of activities were provided by community members [S112]. Several studies reported on community–based HIV testing. One study found that among persons taking antiretroviral therapy, contacts that were visited at home were much more likely to undergo HIV testing than persons seen only at the health clinic [S113]. The prevention of mother–to–child transmission (PMTCT) was the most commonly studied HIV intervention in the assessments reviewed. As PMTCT is discussed in our maternal health paper, only a few examples will be mentioned here. In one study, the probability of survival of children to 18 months of age was 84% higher, compared to those in the control group, when HIV–positive mothers received antiretroviral medication as part of a comprehensive integrated program for HIV exposed infants [S114]. Household visits by CHWs, immunizations and growth monitoring were a part of this project.

The role of household visiting by CHWs was often found to be important for HIV–control projects. In one project, intensive follow–up care by CHWs at the homes of HIV–infected mothers led to much greater compliance with PMTCT and also with antenatal and postnatal care. Initiation of anti–retroviral therapy (ART) for HIV– infected infants was also earlier [S115]. Similarly, CHW home visiting was found to lead to a statistically significant 27% increase in identification of HIV–exposed and infected infants and attendance at health facilities [S116]. Community household visits by midwives who gave counseling and nevirapine to HIV–positive mothers and advised them to give nevirapine to their newborns within 72 hours of birth were found to decrease mother–to–child transmission of HIV by 60% [S117]. Community–based adherence support for 982 children on antiretroviral treatment was found to lead to 60% more children achieving virological suppression than children in the control group ($P = 0.01$) [S118].

In many NGO–led child survival projects included in our review, education about HIV/AIDS with or without PMTCT was part of the project, along with many other interventions, and virtually all of them showed marked increases in knowledge about HIV infection.

Findings specific to immunizations

Immunizations against infectious diseases are well–established as an essential PHC intervention for child health. We have disaggregated the community–based assessments in our database under the areas of activity below.

Promotion and uptake through CHWs or others in routine systems

Community–based interventions involving CHWs reaching to the household level to promote participation in immunization activities and CHWs mobilizing communities have played a key role in producing high rates of population coverage for immunizations throughout the world. Peer education provided by CHWs visiting households, by community members recruited just for this purpose, by female community health education workers, and by members of mobile health teams coming from health facilities have contributed to greatly increased immunization coverage rates for children [S119–123].

Establishment of village networks of trained traditional birth attendants and female CHWs was effective. These CHWs promoted immunizations, use of health facilities, and household diarrhea management with oral rehydration solution (ORS) and also carried out growth monitoring of children. Their activities led to a 150% increase in the coverage of 12–23 month–old children with full immunization [S124].

Village–level approaches to community mobilization

Promotion of community participation through education of village leaders, teachers, and extension workers (who in turn educated community members) was found effective, increasing full immunization completion coverage levels by 50% [S125]. Mass media using TV, radio, newspapers and leaflets, distributed and explained by community–level workers, significantly increased community awareness about immunizations with mothers. Those mothers who had increased awareness were much more likely to take their children to be vaccinated [S126]. In Lao PDR, community–based workshops promoting attendance for vaccination significantly increased all childhood vaccinations [S127].

Promotion of immunizations through microcredit programs

A case–controlled study of community health education campaigns associated with microcredit programs were found to greatly increase fully immunization coverage [S128].

Health Days

National Immunization Days, in which community mobilization and immunization at peripheral service points followed up by immunization at the household for those who did not come to the service point led to significant decreases in the incidence of acute flaccid paralysis [S129]. Annual vaccination weeks with household visits by CHWs increased vaccination completion rates from 30% to 53% [S130].

Household vaccination strategies

A case–controlled study of peer education provided by CHWs visiting households, promoting community involvement, and providing immunizations, vitamin A supplementation and growth monitoring led to not only to greatly increased immunization coverage but also to a 58% decrease in under–5 mortality compared to controls [S131]. House–to–house administration of polio vaccine significantly increased polio vaccination rates [S132].

Findings specific to nutrition

Undernutrition contributes to 45% of under–5 mortality globally [3] and therefore is a major concern. In this section our review findings will be categorized into four areas: protein–energy undernutrition (usually assessed by anthropometry), breastfeeding (BF), complementary feeding (CF), and micronutrient supplementation.

Protein–energy undernutrition

Table 5 presents the findings from randomized controlled and non–randomized controlled studies with statistically significant and operationally large effects compared to controls with protein–energy undernutrition. **Table 5** demonstrates that undernutrition can be addressed successfully at the community level through health education involving CHWs visiting households, regular monitoring of child growth in the community, and supplementation with ready–to–use therapeutic food (RUTF). Albendazole supplementation to mothers also was found to have an important effect on child growth. Even for depressed mothers with HIV, well–organized programs improved the nutrition of their children. Group learning programs associated with small loans (that may have enabled mothers to obtain more nutritious foods for their children) also improved child nutrition. Many other integrated programs were also demonstrated to contribute to good child nutrition. These will be covered below in the final section on integrated programs.

Table 5. Studies of community–based interventions addressing protein energy undernutrition

Intervention	Type of outcome	Population size of study area	Specific outcome	Effect compared to control	Statistical significance	Reference number*
Randomized controlled assessments:						
Home–based distribution of RUTF for children with severe acute, malnutrition	Change in nutritional Status	1178 10–60-mo-old malnourished and wasted children	Attainment of WHZz2 without edema or relapse	Increased by 33%	0.001	[S133]
Education plus micronutrient–fortified milk–based cereal household supplementation	Change in nutritional status	104 infants each in 3 different groups [Supplementation only, counselling only, and control)	Percentage of children with a mean weight gain of 250 g or more	14% more (in supplemental group compared to control group)	0.01	[S134]
Nutrition and hygiene education with growth monitoring at community level	Change in nutritional status	Children 0 to <5 y from 55 randomly selected households	Mean WAZ in older children, mean WAZ in younger children	Increased by 10%; Increased by 36%	0.05; 0.001	[S135]
Albendazole 600 mg every 6 mo provided at household level	Change in nutritional status; morbidity	610 children 18 mo of age who were treated for two years	Prevalence of stunting; prevalence of fecal worms	Decreased by 9%; Decreased by 14%	0.001; 0.001	[S136]
Home visits by CHWs to reduce alcohol use, promote BF, child nutrition, and perinatal HIV regimen compliance	Change in nutritional status	644 depressed mothers and their children 0 to<6 mo	Mean LAZ scores for children 0 to <6 mo	Increased by 7%	0.034	[S137]
Paraprofessional home visits with provision of health education about BF, child nutrition, HIV PMTCT, and mental health	Change in nutritional status	24 township neighborhoods	Mean WHZs for children	Increased by 19%	0.001	[S138]
Non-randomized controlled interventions:						
Home visits from community health agent facilitators to provide education and monthly growth monitoring	Change in nutritional status	14 374 children, 0 to <5 y	Undernutrition in children 0–35 mo	Decreased by 27%	0.05	[S139]
Albendazole 400mg distributed to households with mothers at 12 and 23 weeks of pregnancy	Change in nutritional status	4998 mothers and their children, 0 to<6 mo	Mortality rate in infants during their first 6 mo of life	Decreased by 41%	0.01	[S140]
Using CHWs in a nutritional demonstration (Hearth) program (mothers are trained by participation in cooking nutritious food for children)	Change in nutritional status	1200 children, 3–48 mo	Percentage of children with normal weight for age; percentage of children with severe undernutrition	Increased by 10%; decreased by 18%	0.02; 0.02	[S141], [S141]
Facilitated group learning sessions on maternal and child health with small loans given to mothers	Change in nutritional status	200 children 0 to<3 y	Mean HFA children 12 to 24 mo	Increased by 48%	0.01	[S142]

BF – breastfeeding, HFA – height for age, HIV – human immunodeficiency virus, LAZ – length–for–age Z score, mo – month(s), PMTCT – prevention of mother–to–child transmission, RUTF – ready–to–use–therapeutic food, WHZ – weight–for–height Z score, y – year(s)
*See Appendix S2 in **Online Supplementary Document.**

Other controlled interventions with smaller effect sizes and statistically significant results at the $P < 0.05$ level also were very informative. In Vietnam, among children aged less than 15 months with a weight–for–age Z score of <-2, the Hearth approach along with de–worming significantly improved growth when compared to controls who received only deworming [S143]. The Hearth approach is a process of identifying local "positive deviant" women who have well–nourished children. Mothers of malnourished children are also identified and they are guided through a process of learning how positive deviants care and feed their children and applying this knowledge in the care of their own children through hands–on cooking sessions using locally available foods [S143].

In a non–randomized controlled project that was implemented over a five–year period, the hypothesis was tested that younger siblings of older children with severe undernutrition whose undernutrition had been overcome using the Hearth approach should have better nutrition than similar children whose mothers had not been exposed to the Hearth program. Outcomes were compared for 10 different 3–month age groupings of younger siblings (6–8, 9–11, 12–14, etc.). For younger siblings whose older sibling had been severely malnourished and whose mother had been exposed to the Hearth approach (the intervention group), the younger sibling mean weight for age Z score was always higher than the older sibling ($P = 0.005$ or less in all age groups). For the control group (children with an older sibling who had been moderately malnourished, mildly malnourished, or of normal weight and whose mother had not been exposed to the Hearth program) the same comparison with younger siblings was carried out. The mean weight for age Z score of the younger siblings was always lower for mildly malnourished and normal weight children than their older sibling ($P < 0.05$ for all but one age group, 6–8 months). This study provides evidence regarding the wider family effects of nutritional education [S144]. However any conclusions need to be guarded due to the limited size of the populations studied. These results would need to be repeated in further similar studies.

The benefits of promotion of agriculture and voucher programs on childhood nutrition have also been demonstrated. In a population including 130 000 children younger than 5 years of age in Nepal, promotion of increased household production of food through training Village Model Farmers, and subsequently village women, led over a 2–year period to a decrease of 10% in the prevalence of underweight in children aged 0 to 4 years [S145]. A community development and livestock promotion project in Nepal for 307 children produced similar results. Although the results in the latter study were not statistically significant after 2 years, the intervention group was more likely to have indoor access to water, treat their water and have a latrine. Longer participation in the program was strongly associated with a better mean height–for–age score ($P < 0.00001$) [S146].

Giving vouchers to mothers along with health education and a community household health package was found not to result in statistically significant improved child nutrition in the short term but if the program for those children was extended for 2 years more until the children were aged 8 to 10 years, then the mean height for weight Z scores of these children increased by 23% ($P = 0.029$) compared to controls of the same age [S147]. Other studies demonstrated a statistically significant association of mothers receiving vouchers with greater use of nutrition monitoring at the community level and improved nutrition of their children [S148–151].

Breastfeeding and complementary feeding

Exclusive breastfeeding (BF) during the first 6 months of age with continued BF through the first two years of life is an important contributor to good childhood nutrition, reduced morbidity, and improved mortality in resource–constrained settings. Promotion of exclusive breastfeeding for the first 6 months of life has been estimated to be one of the most effective preventive strategy for saving the lives of young children in low–income settings [9]. Complementary feeding (CF) to supplement breastfeeding is needed from 6 months of age onwards for children to sustain normal growth. Findings from randomized and non–randomized controlled community–based assessments included in our review are presented in **Table 6.**

The data from **Table 6** indicate that exclusive breastfeeding can be effectively promoted at the community level by CHWs, by trained home peer counsellors, by community outreach health professionals from the nearest health facility, and by mothers' community health clubs. Of note is that the strongest effects were found when the CHWs and home peer counselors rather than more highly trained health professionals reaching out from local health facilities were doing the education. Education about complementary feeding was found to produce statistically significant improvements in mean height and weight. The Hearth approach mentioned in the section on protein energy undernutrition was also found to be effective in undernourished children younger than 15 months of age, in the study cited in **Table 5** [S141], and in other studies with similar results [S143, S159, S160].

Table 6. *Community-based projects that promoted breastfeeding and complementary feeding in children*

Intervention	Type of outcome	Population size of study area	Specific outcome	Effect compared to control	Statistical significance	Reference number*
Randomized controlled interventions						
Breastfeeding:						
Training of 1 CHW per village to promote exclusive BF	Change in health-related practice	1115 mothers and their children 0 to <6 mo	Percentage of children exclusively breastfed to <6 mo of age	Increased by 38%	0.05	[S151]
Home counselling by trained CHWs	Change in health-related practice	1597 mothers and their children, 0 to <6 mo	Percentage of children exclusively breastfed to <6 mo of age	Increased by 63%	0.001	[S152]
Home visits by trained women during the postnatal period	Change in health-related practice	175 mothers and their children 0 to <6 mo	Percentage of children exclusively breastfed to <6 mo of age	Increased by 16%	0.001	[S153]
Peer counsellors from community educated pregnant mothers in breastfeeding	Change in health-related practice	726 pregnant women and their children 0 to <6 mo	Exclusive breastfeeding, to <6 mo of age	Increased by 64%	0.01	[S154]
Complementary feeding:						
CHW education of mothers about CF during home visits	Change in nutritional status	118 infants	Prevalence of stunting	Decreased by 10%	<0.05	[S155]
Non–randomized controlled trials:						
Training of mothers in essential nutrition by community outreach workers	Change in health-related practice	320 infants 0 to <6 mo in 8 districts	Percentage of children exclusively breastfed until 6 mo of age	Increased by 22%	0.001	[S156]
Provision of fortified CF at households along with education by CHWs	Change in nutritional status	Children 9–14m in the catchment areas of 10 health clinics	Odds of being underweight after being enrolled in the program for one year	Decreased by 75%	0.007	[S157]
Uncontrolled before–after studies:						
Formation of community health clubs and provision of health education by CHWs	Change in health-related practice	1000 children 0 to <5 y and their mothers	Early initiation of BF; Exclusive BF in children 0–6 mo	Increased by 50%; increased by 60%	0.001; 0.001	[S158], [S158]
Hearth program, CF education by CHWs, nutrition revolving fund established to aid mothers to buy chickens to provide protein for children plus small income	Change in nutritional status	1700 children 0 to <3 y	Prevalence of normal WFA children; prevalence of severe malnutrition	Compared to baseline, increased by 13%; decreased by 17%	0.001; 0.001	[S159], [S159]

3*See Appendix S2 in **Online Supplementary Document.**

Micronutrient supplementation

Types of micronutrient supplementation that were included in projects whose assessments qualified for our review included vitamin A, zinc, iron and multivitamins. **Table 7** contains details about randomized and non–randomized controlled studies that have been included in this review and that have operationally important effects. **Table 7** shows that vitamin A supplementation provided at the household level to mothers, to newborns, and especially to children 6–59 months of age leads to decreased child mortality. Even fortifying market monosodium glutamate with vitamin A leads to a decrease in the rate of xerophthalmia (a condition of eye dryness and eventual scarring produced by vitamin A deficiency) and all–cause child mortality. It also decreases child mortality from pneumonia and measles.

Daily zinc supplementation decreased all–cause mortality in children 12–48 months of age, but not to the same extent as vitamin A. A decrease in the incidence of diarrhea in children receiving zinc has also been demonstrated in other controlled studies [S174, S175]. Of particular note is that in one study of children 1 to <6 months of age in a malaria–prone area, the risk of death or severe morbidity increased significantly in those who received iron supplementation [S176]. While other studies in non–malaria–endemic areas confirmed the value of iron supplementation for treating anemia, this finding provides reason for caution in providing iron supplementation to children aged 1 to <6 months of age in malaria–endemic areas.

Findings specific to integrated approaches to child health

Children present with a variety of common diseases even when one disease such as malaria may predominate in a particular area. Undernutrition is a common risk factor for childhood infections [10,11]. Opportunities to update immunization status need to be taken at every opportunity to prevent serious childhood infections. Mothers may lose confidence in CHWs and CHWs may lose confidence in themselves if CHWs have to turn patients away because they can only deal with one disease entity (or if they do not have the capacity to treat any illnesses). Therefore, for the most cost–effective and efficient use of resources and for increasing the confidence of mothers in CHWs and CHWs in themselves, it is important that services provided be integrated as much as practical for the benefit of all. To do this, a range of integrated approaches have been developed at the community level, and available assessments of the projects have been included in our review.

Table 7. Studies of micronutrient supplementation at the community level

Intervention	Type of outcome	Population size of study area	Specific outcome	Effect compared to control	Statistical significance	Reference number*
Randomized controlled interventions:						
Vitamin A supplementation:						
Supplemental vitamin A 8333 IU weekly and E at the household level	Mortality	7764 children, 0 to <5 y	Risk of death in girls; risk of death in boys	Decreased by 59%; Decreased by 48%	0.01; 0.04	[S161], [S161]
Maternal vitamin A 3330 IU daily and folate supplementation	Mortality	3389 pregnant women and children	Perinatal, and neonatal mortality	Decreased by 20%	0.01	[S162]
Vitamin A (200 000 IU for 12–59 mo–old children, 100 000 IU for 6–11 mo–old children, and 50 000 IU –5m) in a single dose	Mortality	3786 children, 0 to <5 years	1–59 mo mortality	Decreased by 26%	0.05	[S14]
Vitamin A every 4 mo (60 000 IU)	Mortality	28 630 children, 6–72 mo	1–59 mo mortality; case fatality rate for measles	Decreased by 30%; decreased by 76%	0.05; 0.001	[S163], [S163]
Vitamin A 200 000 IU every 6 mo for 18 mo	Morbidity	12 109 children, 9–72 mo	Incidence of night blindness	Decreased by 50%	0.001	[S164]
Vitamin A 200 000 IU for 12–59 mo–old children and 100 000 IU for 1–11m–old children every 4 mo	Mortality	9200 children, 0 to <5 y	1–59 mo mortality	Decreased by 19%	0.05	[S165]
Vitamin A 60 000 IU every 4 mo	Mortality	28 630 children, 6–72 mo	1–59 mo mortality in females	Decreased by 90%	0.0001	[S166]
Vitamin A 200 000 IU for 1–3 mo–old children at 1–3 mo of age and again 6–8 mo later	Mortality	25 000 children, 0 to <5 y	1–59 mo mortality	Decreased by 34%	0.01	[S167]
Infants received 24 000 IU of vitamin A on days 1 and 2 after delivery	Mortality	5786 newborns	Mortality during the 1st 6m of life	Decreased by 22%	0.02	[S168]
Vitamin A given at birth (50 000 IU)	Mortality	7953 newborns	All–cause infant mortality	Decreased by 15%	0.045	[S169]
Vitamin A 200 000 IU for 12–59 mo–old children and 100 000 IU for 1–11 mo–old infants	Morbidity	1405 children, 6–47 mo	Incidence of acute respiratory infection in normal children.	Increased by 8%	0.05	[S170]
Vitamin A 200 000 IU for 12–59 mo–old children and 100 000 IU for 1–11 mo– old infants twice a year and accompanied by nutrition education	Change in nutritional status	720 children 0–36 mo	Prevalence of stunting	Decreased by 11%	0.01	[S171]
Zinc supplementation:						
Vitamin A 200 000 IU as one dose plus 10 mg zinc 6 days a week	Morbidity	148 children, 6–72 mo	Prevalence of malaria	Decreased by 32%	<0.001	[S172]
Zinc (70 mg) weekly for one year	Morbidity	809 children, 6–18 mo	Incidence of pneumonia	Decreased by 44%	0.01	[S83]

Table 7. *Continued*

Intervention	Type of outcome	Population size of study area	Specific outcome	Effect compared to control	Statistical significance	Reference number*
Daily supplementation with 10 mg of zinc	Mortality	21 274 children, 12–48 mo for 485 days	Relative risk of all-cause mortality in children 12–48 mo	Decreased by 18%	0.045	[S173]
Daily supplementation with 10 mg of zinc	Morbidity	854 children 6–48 mo	Incidence of diarrhea in children 0 to <2 y	Decreased by 25%	0.001	[S174]
Zinc 20mg zinc daily for 15 d (for children with diarrhea)	Morbidity	139 children 6–35 mo	Duration of persistent diarrhea	Decreased by 28%	0.01	[S175]
Iron supplementation:						
Iron, folate and zinc supplementation: iron (12.5 mg), folic acid (5 µg) zinc (10mg) daily	Morbidity	Children, 1 to <6 mo	Risk of severe morbidity (from severe malaria) and death in groups that received iron	Increased by 12%	0.02	[S176]
Sale to households of "Sprinkles" (a powder to sprinkle on top of food) containing iron and B vitamins	Morbidity	561 children, 0 to <5 y	Prevalence of anemia	Decreased by 19%	0.001	[S177]
Daily home fortification with micronutrient powder containing iron for 2 mo	Change in nutritional status	1103 children, 0 to <5 y	Mean hemoglobin concentration	Increased by 7%	0.001	[S178]
Multivitamin and mineral powder (MMP) supplement: 2 sachets 2 times a week (compared to 2 sachets MMP daily and controls)	Morbidity	115 children, 0 to <5 y in each of the 3 groups	Prevalence of anemia, compliance with MMP supplement	Decreased by 32% in daily MMP; 200% greater in 2 times a week group compared to daily	0.001; 0.001	[S179]
Non-randomized controlled interventions:						
Vitamin A supplementation:						
Fortification of monosodium gluconate sold in markets with vitamin A	Morbidity	5755 children 0 to <5 y	Prevalence of Bitot's spots; mortality	Decreased by 600%; mortality rate among pre-school children in the control villages was 1.8 times greater than that for children in intervention villages	0.0001; 0.001	[S180], [S180]
Education on weaning practices, Vitamin A provision to children, Provision of iron to mothers, immunization, door-to-door visits from CHWs	Mortality	6663 children, 0–35 mo and 14 551 women	All-cause mortality among children 6–35 mo; pneumonia-specific mortality among children 6–35 mo	Decreased by 32%; decreased by 53%	0.001; 0.001	[S181], [S181]

Integrated Management of Childhood Illness (IMCI) and Integrated Community Case Management (iCCM)

Integrated Management of Childhood Illness (IMCI) integrates the prevention and treatment of all childhood illness at health facilities. Its community component, called Community IMCI (or C–IMCI), usually consists of preventive activities and early recognition of potentially serious acute illness that can be performed in the community by trained CHWs going door–to–door and meeting with groups, usually without treatment of illnesses other than ORS for diarrhea. CHWs are taught to recognize children with danger signs and refer or even escort patients to the nearest health facility for treatment. CHWs also facilitate outreach activities from the local health center such as immunizations.

Integrated Community Case Management (iCCM) enables CHWs to diagnose and treat serious acute illnesses of childhood (acute respiratory infection, diarrhea, malaria and in some cases acute malnutrition).

For iCCM to be effective, CHWs need to be well–trained, to have the confidence and support of their community, to be well–linked to their local health facility staff for referral of patients, to receive regular supervision to maintain their skills, and to be well–supplied with the drugs and equipment necessary to perform their tasks [12]. These CHWs often also have community health education roles, perform household visiting, and may also be responsible for such activities as promotion and distribution of ITNs. Studies of IMCI and iCCM are often concerned with maintaining the quality of all the above tasks. **Table 8** summarizes the findings of assessments of C–IMCI and iCCM interventions. The studies described in **Table 8** show that iCCM can be implemented successfully at the community level and indeed may lead to a decrease in under–5 mortality. A large assessment of children younger than 5 years of age in 15 districts in Rwanda with complete mortality data further supports this. This assessment found that the number of children receiving community–based treatment for diarrhea and pneumonia increased significantly in the 1–year period after iCCM implementation, from 0.83 cases/1000 child–months to 3.80 cases/1000 child–months ($P < 0.001$) and from 0.25 cases/1000 child–months to 5.28 cases/1000 child–months ($P < 0.001$), respectively. On average, total under–5 mortality rates declined significantly by 38% ($P < 0.001$), and health facility use declined significantly by 15%. These decreases were significantly greater than expected based on baseline trends [S192].

In many parts of rural Uganda with limited access to trained health staff, up to 50% of cases of childhood illnesses are managed by drug sellers. One study in which private drug sellers were trained to treat patients using iCCM

Table 8. *Studies of the effectiveness of Community–Integrated Management of Childhood Illnesses (C–IMCI) and Integrated Community Case Management (iCCM)*

Intervention	Type of outcome	Population size of study area	Specific outcome	Effect compared to control	Statistical significance	Reference number*
Randomized controlled trials:						
CHWs trained as part of the family and community activities associated with IMCI, as well as health system strengthening	Mortality; change in nutritional status	The catchment areas of 10 health facilities (175 000 persons)	All–cause mortality 0 to <5 y; prevalence of exclusive breast feeding 0 to <6 mo	Decreased by 13.4%; Increased by 10.1%	0.01; 0.05	[S182]
Non-randomized controlled trials:						
Linkage of CHWs with local health facilities and provision of training to CHWs	Coverage; change in nutritional status	Children 0 to <2 y in a population of 160 000	Percentage of children 12–23 mo fully immunized; percentage of children receiving at least five meals per day	Increased by 21%; increased by 32%	0.05; 0.05	[S183]
Awareness seminars conducted during the first year for leaders of all villages followed 1 y later by similar seminars for extension workers and teachers	Coverage; change in nutritional status	Women of child–bearing age and their children in villages with a total population of 18 000	Percentage of children with full immunization coverage; percentage of children with severe undernutrition	Increased by 50%; decreased by 27%	0.001; 0.05	[S184]
CHWs trained in iCCM	Mortality	Children <5 y in villages with a total population of 14 000	Under–5 mortality	Decreased by 38%	0.003	[S185]
On–site monthly supervision on C–IMCI by trained supervisors of Health Extension Workers (HEWs)	Quality of care	500 HEWs assessed	Quality of case management over two years (percentage of cases that were correctly classified, treated, and followed–up within two days of initiating treatment)	Increased by 200%	0.04	[S186]
C–IMCI with 2 HEWs working at a community health post	Quality of care	87 HEWS	Correct prescription of anti–malarial medications in comparison to HEWs working in a vertical malaria control program	Increased by 10%	0.05	[S187]
Drug sellers trained in iCCM protocols	Quality of care	Sick children who made 7667 visits to 44 trained drug sellers	Correct treatment of common illnesses	Increased by 27%	0.001	[S188]

Table 8. *Continued*

Intervention	Type of outcome	Population size of study area	Specific outcome	Effect compared to control	Statistical significance	Reference number*
Peer support groups among CHWs trained in iCCM	Coverage	1575 children in 6 districts	Number of sick children treated for ARI, malaria, and diarrhea (compared to CHWs trained in iCCM without peer support groups)	Increased by 167%	0.001	[S189]
CHWs trained in iCCM	Coverage	306 190 children 6 mo to <5 y	Number of sick children treated for ARI, malaria, diarrhea	Increased by 23%	0.05	[S190]
CHWs trained in iCCM	Coverage	38 009 children <5 y	Percentage of children sleeping under ITNS	Increased by 33%	0.01	[S191]

ARI – acute respiratory infection, HEW – health extension workers, ITN – insecticide-treated bed nets, mo – month(s), y – year(s)
*See Appendix S2 in **Online Supplementary Document**.

protocols revealed a strong adherence to the iCCM protocol in terms of testing, examining and treating children. On follow up evaluation after training, 88% of children diagnosed with diarrhea received ORS. 88% of children presenting with a fever received a RDT for malaria and 94% of children who were diagnosed as RDT–positive received artemisinin combination therapy. Of those who were diagnosed with pneumonia, 91% of them received amoxicillin treatment. Overall performance (defined as correct treatment) showed a 27% ($P = 0.001$) increase compared with baseline levels [S188]. The other studies cited in **Table 8** demonstrate that monthly community–level supervision by trained supervisors from the local health facility can lead to maintenance of CHW skills in iCCM diagnosis and treatment and that iCCM leads to more children receiving treatment for these common illnesses [S186, S189–191].

Care Groups

Care Groups were included in the review through the publication of the results of the evaluation of several projects. A Care Group is a group of 10–15 community volunteers who act as community–based health educators. The Care Group meets every two weeks with a project facilitator for two hours or so to learn some new education messages. Each volunteer is responsible for regularly visiting

10–15 of her neighbors, sharing the new messages they just learned. With this structure and basic approach, scaling up is readily possible [13,14].

In a 5–year Care Group project in Sofala Province in Mozambique, the project area was divided into two sub–areas (A and B) since project activities began several years later in Area B after activities in Area A had begun. Major improvements were achieved across most indicators of child health comparing baseline with endline findings. Key outcomes were that the overall proportion of children with undernutrition (WAZ<–2.0 SD) decreased by 6% in Area A and by 10% in Area B; insecticide–treated bed net (ITN) use increased by 45% in Area A and by 71% in Area B; rates of exclusive breastfeeding increased by 60% in Area A and 25% in Area B; the percentage of children 9–23m of age who ate three or more meals per day increased from by 42% in Area A and by 20% in Area B. Based on findings obtained with the Lives Saved Tool (LiST), the project saved an estimated 6848 lives and the cost per life saved, the cost per disability–adjusted life year (DALY) averted, and the annual cost per beneficiary were US$ 441, US$ 14.72 and US $2.78, respectively [S193].

Another Care Group project in the rural part of the Chokwe District in Mozambique also incorporated a community–based vital events registry system as part of the activities of the Care Groups. The assessment of this project demonstrated not only the efficacy of Care Groups but also the quality of a community–based vital events registration system. This assessment demonstrated that the Care Group approach resulted in a 49% decrease in the infant mortality rate and a 42% decrease in the under–5 mortality rate over the five year period of project implementation, confirmed by an independent retrospective morality assessment based on maternal birth histories [S194]. Similar results were found in another Care Group project in our database in Burundi [S195].

Integrated community–based primary health care (CBPHC)

Primary health care (PHC) includes the provision of a comprehensive range of essential preventive and treatment actions aimed at meeting all the common health needs of community members (especially those of women of childbearing age and children but also of men and older women) using practical and affordable approaches. For integrated CBPHC to be effective at the community level outside of health facilities, CHWs need to have good linkages to the local health facility to which patients with severe illness, injuries and uncommon or more severe illnesses can be referred and where mothers can give birth. Services such as immunizations that require outreach from health facilities also need to be provided at the community level in order to make essential services readily available. Our review includes a number of community–based PHC programs that are presented in **Table 9**.

Table 9 demonstrates that primary health care with strong community–based components can decrease under–5 mortality. Promotion of community involvement and training/deployment of CHWs is also shown to be a recurring element of these successful programs. Assessments S196–198 are three studies from the Navrongo experiment in Ghana. In the Navrongo experiment in Ghana, there were four groups compared: (1) community health nurses alone–called Community Health Officers, (2) community volunteers and community mobilization without community health nurses; (3) both community health nurses and community volunteers with community mobilization, and (4) a control group. The group that only had community volunteers did not reduce child mortality but did significantly improve child nutrition [S196]. The community–based nurses provided curative care and were effective in decreasing child mortality but did not improve child nutrition or contraceptive coverage [S197]. The best results were achieved when nurses worked with community volunteers and mobilized community members improving child mortality, child nutrition and contraceptive use, together with a 15% improvement in contraceptive coverage [S198].

The census–based, impact–oriented (CBIO) methodology includes mapping and community registering to ensure that all beneficiaries are documented and included in the project information system so that they are included in all community–based PHC programs [S200, S201]. The CBIO approach was pioneered in Haiti in the 1970s. Assessment by retrospective maternal birth histories and household anthropometric surveys demonstrated a 68% reduction in under–5 mortality and reduced prevalence of stunting compared to national rural indicators [S202, S203].

The last assessment in **Table 9** is the earliest one in our database and was reported in 1951 [S204]. It was carried out at a time when there had not yet been many experiences with CHWs and when CHWs were used only for health promotion and referral for provision of health services at a health center.

One important study in our database that does not lend itself to incorporation into **Table 9** is the Narangwal Project, which pioneered many elements of CBPHC [S205]. It operated from 1967 to 1973 in the rural Punjab of Northern India. The nutrition and health–care aspects of this study are of direct relevance to CBPHC and child health. There were four cells in the nutrition aspect of this non–randomized controlled study: (A) a nutrition–only cell, (B) a health–care–only cell, (C) a combined nutrition–and–health–care cell, and (D) a control cell

Table 9. *Primary health care programs that have strong community–based components*

Intervention	Type of outcome	Population size of study area	Specific outcome	Effect compared to control	Statistical significance	Reference number*
Randomized controlled assessments:						
PHC with full range of child health services provided by CHWs plus outreach services.	Change in nutritional status	788 children 6–23 mo	Height–for–age Z score, Weight–for–age Z score	Increased by 24%, increased by 14%	0.018, 0.05	[S196]
PHC nurses posted in communities without CHWs	Mortality	2000 children <5 y	Under–5 mortality	Decreased by 54%	0.05	[S197]
PHC promoting community involvement with volunteer CHWs and well–trained Community Health Officers	Mortality	51 407 children <5 y	Mortality of children exposed to intervention for more than 2 y	Decreased by 60%	0.001	[S198]
PHC with full range of child health services provided by CHWs plus outreach services	Mortality	6663 children 0–35 mo, 14 551 women	All–cause mortality in children 6–35 mo. Pneumonia–specific mortality in children 6–35 mo	Decreased by 32%. Decreased by 53%.	0.001	[S199]
Non–randomized controlled assessments:						
Census–based PHC with frequent visits by CHWs to all households, distribution of vitamin A, provision of growth monitoring, education, immunizations, and transport assistance when referral needed	Mortality	15 406 (total population of intervention area)	All–cause under–5 mortality	Decreased by 52%	0.001	[S200]
Peer education, referral, and promotion of community involvement in planning, implementing, and evaluating services provided by volunteer CHWs	Mortality	36 000 children <5 y	All–cause under–5 mortality	Decreased by 58%	0.0001	[S201]
PHC with outreach, health education, supplemental feeding, immunizations, curative treatment, TB control, support of TBAs	Mortality	2700 children aged 0–6 y	All–cause under–5 mortality; stunting	Decreased by 67%; reduced by 28% in children 48–59m	0.0001, 0.001	[S202], [S203]
PHC provided at a health center with community outreach by trained health assistants	Mortality	887 persons in health center catchment area	Crude mortality of all age groups over a time period of 10 y until 1951	Decreased by 24%	0.001	[S204]

CHW – community health worker, mo – month(s), PHC – primary health care, TBA – traditional birth attendant, y – year(s)
*Appendix S2 in **Online Supplementary Document**.

(in which routine government services without outreach were provided). Promotion of community participation was a key aspect of the design of this study. Each cell contained approximately 200–300 children. Child nutrition services included growth monitoring and promotion as well as food supplementation twice daily. The child health care services included infectious disease surveillance and early treatment, immunizations, and education concerning disease prevention. In the nutrition study, mortality rates were significantly reduced during the perinatal, neonatal, post–neonatal, and 12–23 month age groups in both the nutrition cell as well as in the nutrition + health care cell compared to the control cell. In addition, the weight–for–age and height–for–age of children beyond 17 months of age were significantly greater in the nutrition cell and in the nutrition + health care cell compared to control cell [S205].

Key CBPHC aspects of this project were that Family Health Workers provided treatment in the home for dehydration from diarrhea and for childhood pneumonia. The children 0–3 years of age with pneumonia who were treated with penicillin had a 42% reduced risk of overall mortality [S206]. Other key findings based on a qualitative review of data were that: one–on–one education of mothers was essential for improving practices related to breastfeeding, infant feeding, rehydration and feeding of sick infants and also for overcoming traditional beliefs about not feeding a child with diarrhea; weekly home visits were necessary in order to achieve a reduction in infant mortality; delegation of services as far to the periphery as possible improved coverage and effectiveness; rehabilitation of malnourished children through special feeding programs was best accomplished at home or near the home; having a curative health care service was an essential element of building trust, and developing a quality health care program required active community participation and building trust with the community [S207].

Several other assessments included in our database are of particular note since they document the evidence of the long–term benefits of CBPHC projects on child health. These projects are:

- The ICDDR,B MCH–FP Program in Matlab, Bangladesh (a maternal/child health and family planning research field site for the International Centre for Diarrheal Disease Research, Bangladesh/Centre for Health, Population and Nutrition);
- The Hôpital Albert Schweitzer in Deschapelles, Haiti;
- The Jamkhed Comprehensive Health Project in Jamkhed, India; and,
- SEARCH (Society for Education, Action and Research in Community Health) in Gadchiroli, India.

These projects are discussed in detail elsewhere in this supplement [15].

DISCUSSION

This review provides strong evidence that overall the major causes of child mortality in developing countries can be addressed at the community level outside of health facilities by working with communities and community–level workers. For all categories of interventions, we have presented findings from randomized and non–randomized controlled trials in our database that have consistently produced statistically significant and operationally important effects. In many cases the outcomes observed have been changes in the most objective and meaningful indicator: mortality.

Some assessments, mostly unpublished child survival project evaluations, relied on before/after study designs without a comparison group, measuring changes in population coverage of key child survival interventions. In virtually all cases, the changes in coverage over a 4–5 year period were quite pronounced, particularly in comparison to much smaller changes in coverage in the regional or national population, as a review of a set of these projects has demonstrated [16]. They have generally produced statistically significant and operationally important results. Other less rigorous assessments of the effectiveness of CBPHC in improving child health were not included in this article due to space limitations, but they also provide evidence supporting our major findings presented here.

Our findings regarding the effectiveness of specific community–based interventions for improving child health are similar to those reported in other reviews [4,17]. The provision of iron to children in malaria–endemic areas, whether through community–based approaches or otherwise, may have harmful effects so it not recommended at this time. However, this is the only evidence we have identified in which implementation of CBPHC intervention led to a less than favorable effect. However, it is important to note that this finding pertains to the biomedical interaction of iron on children exposed to malaria rather than on the effectiveness of CBPHC as a strategy for improving child health. At the community level the total number of interventions being implemented – even in a comprehensive primary health care approach – may be spread amongst several CHWs working in a team each of whom may do only one or two interventions. Consequently, evidence about the effectiveness of one or two interventions implemented by individuals, usually CHWs, is consistent with "community–based primary health care."

We have not addressed here three important questions: (1) who are the community–level workers who implemented the interventions, (2) what particular resources do they need in order to deliver the interventions, and (3) what are the conditions that would need to be met in order to scale up these interventions under routine conditions. Answering these questions is beyond the scope of this paper, and few assessments really address these questions, unfortunately. The degree to which the assessments included here represent efficacy studies (that is, project implementation under ideal field conditions) as opposed to effectiveness studies (implementation under routine field conditions) cannot be adequately explored here. However, it is clear that appropriately trained, supervised and supported CHWs along with engaged communities are needed to achieve effectiveness, and these conditions appear to have been met in the projects included in our review.

This review demonstrates that four major strategies for delivering community–based primary health care interventions are effective and commonly used in projects that have improved child health. These strategies are (1) house–to–house visitation by CHWs; (2) community case management of childhood illness, (3) use of participatory women's groups; and (4) outreach services provided in the community by mobile teams based at peripheral health centers. CHWs visit households to educate child caregivers about prevention and manage common illnesses. Through following well–developed protocols, CHWs link community members to their nearest health facility for management of serious illness or follow up. These strategies are discussed in detail elsewhere in this series from the perspective of CBPHC strategies for improving maternal, neonatal as well as child health [18].

Many assessments included in our review support the importance of community engagement. A systematic review of child survival programs has found that programs working collaboratively with the community can lead to cost–effective transformation and lasting behavior change that produces improved health outcomes [19]. As a result of such engagements, the knowledge that community members have about what works locally is more likely to be shared with health program staff because they have a shared responsibility for program planning, implementation and evaluation. Without being a stakeholder, community members may see programs as imposed from the outside and not responsive to their needs. Without community engagement, programs may not produce the best outcomes that might otherwise be achieved through strong community engagement.

While we have made every effort to include all relevant studies that meet our criteria, some important studies have escaped our screening process. One such study concerns the use of pre–referral rectal artesunate [20]. In a randomized controlled trial in Bangladesh, Ghana and Tanzania, patients aged 6 to 72 months with suspected severe malaria who could not be treated orally were allocated randomly to receive a single rectal dose of artesunate (n = 8954) or placebo (n = 8872) before referral to a clinic where antimalarial injections could be given. In patients who had not reached a clinic within 6 hours, half of whom had not reached a clinic within 15 hours, pre–referral artesunate significantly reduced death or permanent disability by half (1.9% in the intervention group compared to 3.8% in the control group).

Several studies included in our review confirmed the effectiveness of Integrated Community Case Management (iCCM) (**Table 8**). However, several recent evaluations published since the end–point of publications selected for our review (31 December 2015) have found that iCCM, when implemented at scale, has not expanded coverage of key child survival interventions or reduced under–5 mortality, partly because of shortcomings related to training, supervision and drug stock outs [21] and low levels of care seeking [22,23]. Perhaps CHWs trained in iCCM are not able to make frequent home visits and therefore unable to give sufficient attention to educating mothers about warning signs for which they should seek care or to earn their confidence. Their broader job responsibilities beyond iCCM, including providing curative care for adults and family planning for women, as well as the large size of their catchment areas (sometimes more than 2 hours away from their health post) make frequent home visits virtually impossible.

As the Narangwal project demonstrated four decades ago, the provision of some curative care builds community trust in the CHWs providing it. It also facilitates referral to local health facilities as needed. However this trust is difficult to develop if the CHWs are not in regular contact with all households and if community members are not convinced that the CHWs are well trained and competent. One particularly important recent example of the effectiveness achieved by meeting these conditions occurred in Yirimadjo, Mali [S93]. The intervention included CHW active case finding, user fee removal, infrastructure development, community mobilization and prevention programming. After three years of the intervention, the hazard of under–5 mortality in the intervention area was one tenth that of baseline (HR 0.10 $P < 0.0001$), the prevalence of febrile illness of children younger than 5 years of age was significantly lower, from 38% at baseline to 23% at endline ($P = 0.0009$) and the percentage of children starting an effective antimalarial with 24 hours of symptom onset was nearly twice that reported at baseline ($P = 0.0195$).

The assessments from the Navrongo project in Ghana [S196–198] demonstrate that the best results were achieved when the community nurses worked in conjunction with trained community volunteers and community mobilization. The particular processes of community mobilization focused on working through the traditional community structure and engaging persons with a leadership role within the community. While the community–based nurses did have some impact on child mortality through their provision of prompt curative treatment, they did not have significant impact on contraceptive use or on child nutrition that require a high level of trust between community members and providers that can be achieved by community participation and door–to–door provision of support and health education [24]. A more recent evaluation of the extension of this program across Ghana indicates that an ongoing systematic approach with regular planning, monitoring and supervision of health workers, and close collaboration with community leaders needs to be followed to produce lasting results at scale [25].

For CBPHC to be most effective it must reach all households, including the poorest families, all mothers, those households far away, and those who are members of religious or ethnic minorities. In our review, the census–based, impact–oriented (CBIO) approach and Care Groups have demonstrated the importance of registering and visiting frequently all households with mothers and children, as more recent evidence has also demonstrated [26,27] . The Care Group approach has achieved excellent results at low cost [14] and is currently being implemented in many priority countries [13].

The following essential interventions for child health that can be provided at the level of the community and/or health post by CHWs have been identified [1]:

- Promote breastfeeding (including exclusive breastfeeding during the first six months of life) and appropriate complementary feeding beginning at 6 months of age
- Provide vitamin A and zinc supplementation
- Provide co–trimoxazole for HIV–positive children
- Educate families on safe disposal of children's stools and hand washing
- Distribute and promote use of ITNs or IRs or both
- Detect and refer children with severe acute malnutrition
- Prevent, diagnose and treat pneumonia of pneumonia, malaria and diarrheal diseases with early referral of those children with danger signs of serious disease.

The strong and consistent evidence that we have presented in this paper clearly demonstrates that all these Essential Interventions can be delivered at the community level with favorable population–level results for children.

The findings from this review also provide strong evidence that the four key strategies of delivering community–based interventions are effective approaches for achieving implementation effectiveness through CBPHC. These strategies are: (1) house–to–house visitation by CHWs; (2) community case management of childhood illness, (3) use of participatory women's groups; and (4) outreach services provided in the community by mobile teams based at health centers. We have also presented evidence that community participation and mobilization make a strong contribution to intervention effectiveness.

Study limitations

Some of the studies included in our review lacked sufficient information about the assessment methodology, about the role of community members and other implementation strategies, as well as about the outcomes themselves. This sometimes made it difficult to assess the strength of the evidence and to draw firm conclusions. We worked to mitigate this limitation by, in some cases, following up with the authors of these assessments.

Due to space limitations not all 489 assessments of the effectiveness of CB-PHC in improving child health could be cited in this analysis. However, the findings of the assessments not specifically cited here are consistent with and supportive of those that were cited.

As is well–known, project failures and serious challenges encountered in program implementation are rarely described in open–access documents or in the scientific literature. This means that a serious publication bias is present and should be recognized. Nonetheless, publication bias does not negate the value of the numerous assessments that have been included in our review that demonstrate effectiveness of CBPHC in improving child health. The consistency of findings across many assessments in relationship to most interventions is such that we are convinced that the general findings with respect to each specific intervention are valid.

We acknowledge that there may be some assessments that qualified for our review that were not picked up by our screening procedures. However, we do not think that the inclusion of any articles we might have missed would alter the overall findings from our review. In addition, we are aware that there are important findings in papers published after December 2015 that did not fit the timeline of our review, but we have highlighted them in the discussion.

Our review has identified several areas of further study that are needed to address gaps in current knowledge to improve the implementation of child health programs at the community level. These areas are:

- Effectiveness studies of the implementation of community based interventions at scale in large populations in routine settings for 5 or more years;

- Effectiveness studies on how best to involve communities in the monitoring, implementation and evaluation of these settings.

As can be readily seen from the tables in this paper there is a clear lack of assessments of studies of interventions in large populations at scale. In the final paper of this series [28] the Expert Panel highlights the need for more evidence from programs delivered at scale. Similarly, while we have provided evidence that many interventions can be implemented successfully at the community level, the actual results produced in the field depend on how well community members "own" and therefore use the interventions provided in a sustainable manner. How to best do this needs further investigation.

Given the heterogeneity of (1) the types of interventions implemented, (2) the manner in which they were implemented, and (3) the outcome measures used to assess outcomes, it is not possible to make any definitive statements about the strength of the evidence or the magnitude of effect for any specific intervention or any specific approach to implementation, or how any given intervention or implementation approach compares with another in terms of effectiveness. Moreover, addressing the important issue of how to most effectively integrate interventions into a balanced package of services so that the demands for implementation of one intervention do not override the requirements for implementation of another intervention is beyond the scope of this paper, as is the important issue of how to strengthen health systems more broadly to better support the implementation of effective CBPHC interventions for improving child health.

Nonetheless, consistent with the purpose of our overall review of the effectiveness of CBPHC in improving MNCH, our overall findings strongly support the conclusion that (1) CBPHC can in fact be effectively implemented at the community level to improve child health and (2) robust community–based delivery systems are needed in order for the evidence–based interventions currently known and those that will be developed can reach their full potential.

CONCLUSIONS

We have presented the evidence of effectiveness of a broad range of community–based interventions for improving the health of children 1–59 months of age. Health systems that are capable of achieving universal coverage of these interventions in high–mortality settings are clearly needed. Achieving this capability will require strong support for the health system as well as a strong commitment to a well–trained and well–supported CHW cadre in sufficient numbers. Understanding the conditions that need to be met in order for these interventions to be effective at scale in routine settings in priority countries and ensuring that these conditions are met will be the major challenge in the decade to come.

Acknowledgements: *The authors wish to thank Zulfi Bhutta for comments on earlier drafts of this manuscript, and the many students and research assistants who contributed to the assembling the database and the analysis. We are grateful to the following organizations that provided small grants to cover the expenses of this review: UNICEF, the World Bank, the Department of Child and Adolescent Health and Development of the World Health Organization, the CORE Group (Collaboration and Resources for Child Health)/ USAID, Future Generations, and the Gates Foundation. We are also grateful to the American Public Health Association and particularly its International Health Section staff, which administered some of these funds. We thank Future Generations for providing office space, administrative support, and salary support to Dr Perry during the initial phase of the review. The World Bank made it possible for one of its consultants, Dr Bahie Rassekh, to participate as a member of the Study Team.*

Funding: *The following organizations provided funds that were used to conduct the work described in this article: The World Health Organization, UNICEF, the World Bank, the United States Agency for International Development, and the Gates Foundation. The organizations that provided financial support had no role in the execution of the review.*

Authorship declaration: *PF wrote the first draft. All of the authors participated in the revision of earlier drafts and approved the final draft.*

Conflict of interest: *All authors have completed the Unified Competing Interest Form at www.icmje.org/coi_disclosure.pdf (available upon request from the corresponding author), and declare no conflict of interest.*

References

1 Black RE, Levin C, Walker N, Chou D, Liu L, Temmerman M, et al. Reproductive, maternal, newborn, and child health: key messages from Disease Control Priorities 3rd Edition. Lancet. 2016;388:2811-24.

2 Liu L, Johnson HL, Cousens S, Perin J, Scott S, Lawn JE, et al. Global, regional, and national causes of child mortality: an updated systematic analysis for 2010 with time trends since 2000. Lancet. 2012;379:2151-61. Medline:22579125 doi:10.1016/S0140-6736(12)60560-1

3 Black RE, Victora CG, Walker SP, Bhutta ZA, Christian P, de Onis M, et al. Maternal and child undernutrition and overweight in low-income and middle-income countries. Lancet. 2013;382:427-51. Medline:23746772 doi:10.1016/S0140-6736(13)60937-X

4 Lassi ZS, Kumar R, Bhutta ZA. Community-based care to improve maternal, newborn, and child health. 2016. In: Disease Control Priorities: Reproductive, Maternal, Newborn, and Child Health, Third Edition. Washington, DC: World Bank, Available: https:// openknowledge.worldbank.org/bitstream/handle/10986/23833/9781464803482. pdf?sequence=3&isAllowed=y. Accessed: 20 March 2017.

5 Perry H, Rassekh B, Gupta S, Wilhelm J, Freeman P. A comprehensive review of the evidence regarding the effectiveness of community-based primary health care in improving maternal, neonatal and child health: 1. rationale, methods and database description. J Glob Health. 2017;07:010901.

6 Jennings M, Pradhan S, Schleiff M, Sacks E, Freeman P, Gupta S, et al. A comprehensive review of the evidence regarding the effectiveness of community-based primary health care in improving maternal, neonatal and child health: 2. maternal health findings. J Glob Health. 2017;7:010902.

7 Sacks E, Freeman P, Sakyi K, Jennings M, Rassekh B, Gupta S, et al. A comprehensive review of the evidence regarding the effectiveness of community-based primary health care in improving maternal, neonatal and child health: 3. neonatal health findings. J Glob Health. 2017;7:010903.

8 WHO. UNICEF. ending preventable child deaths from pneumonia and diarrhoea by 2025. The integrated Global Action Plan for Pneumonia and Diarrhoea (GAPPD). 2013. Available: http://www.unicef.org/immunization/files/GAPPD.pdf. Accessed: 20 March 2017.

9 Jones G, Steketee RW, Black RE, Bhutta ZA, Morris SS. How many child deaths can we prevent this year? Lancet. 2003;362:65-71. Medline:12853204 doi:10.1016/S0140-6736(03)13811-1

10 Pelletier DL, Frongillo EA Jr, Schroeder DG, Habicht JP. The effects of malnutrition on child mortality in developing countries. Bull World Health Organ. 1995;73:443-8. Medline:7554015

11 Caulfield LE, de Onis M, Blossner M, Black RE. Undernutrition as an underlying cause of child deaths associated with diarrhea, pneumonia, malaria, and measles. Am J Clin Nutr. 2004;80:193-8. Medline:15213048

12 Bosch-Capblanch X, Marceau C. Training, supervision and quality of care in selected integrated community case management (iCCM) programmes: a scoping review of programmatic evidence. J Glob Health. 2014;4:020403. Medline:25520793 doi:10.7189/jogh.04.020403

13 Perry H, Morrow M, Borger S, Weiss J, DeCoster M, Davis T, et al. Care Groups I: an innovative community-based strategy for improving maternal, neonatal, and child health in resource-constrained settings. Glob Health Sci Pract. 2015;3:358-69. Medline:26374798 doi:10.9745/GHSP-D-15-00051

14 Perry H, Morrow M, Davis T, Borger S, Weiss J, DeCoster M, et al. Care Groups II: a summary of the maternal, neonatal and child health outcomes achieved in high-mortality, resource-constrained settings. Glob Health Sci Pract. 2015;3:370-81. Medline:26374799 doi:10.9745/GHSP-D-15-00052

15 Perry H, Rassekh B, Gupta S, Freeman P. A comprehensive review of the evidence regarding the effectiveness of community-based primary health care in improving maternal, neonatal and child health: 7. programs with evidence of long-term impact on mortality in children younger than five years of age. J Glob Health. 2017;7:010907.

16 Ricca J, Kureshy N, Leban K, Prosnitz D, Ryan L. Community-based intervention packages facilitated by NGOs demonstrate plausible evidence for child mortality impact. Health Policy Plan. 2014;29:204-16. Medline:23434515 doi:10.1093/heapol/czt005

17 Bhutta ZA, Das JK, Rizvi A, Gaffey MF, Walker N, Horton S, et al. Evidence-based interventions for improvement of maternal and child nutrition: what can be done and at what cost? Lancet. 2013;382:452-77. Medline:23746776 doi:10.1016/S0140-6736(13)60996-4

18 Perry H, Rassekh B, Gupta S, Freeman P. A comprehensive review of the evidence regarding the effectiveness of community-based primary health care in improving maternal, neonatal and child health: 6. strategies used by effective projects. J Glob Health. 2017;7:010906.

19 Farnsworth SK, Bose K, Fajobi O, Souza PP, Peniston A, Davidson LL, et al. Community engagement to enhance child survival and early development in low- and middle-income countries: an evidence review. J Health Commun. 2014;19 Suppl 1:67-88. Medline:25207448 doi:10.1080/10810730.2014.941519

20 Gomes MF, Faiz MA, Gyapong JO, Warsame M, Agbenyega T, Babiker A, et al. Pre-referral rectal artesunate to prevent death and disability in severe malaria: a placebo-controlled trial. Lancet. 2009;373:557-66. Medline:19059639 doi:10.1016/S0140-6736(08)61734-1

21 Munos M, Guiella G, Roberton T, Maiga A, Tiendrebeogo A, Tam Y, et al. Independent evaluation of the rapid scale-up program to reduce under-five mortality in Burkina Faso. Am J Trop Med Hyg. 2016;94:584-95. Medline:26787147 doi:10.4269/ajtmh.15-0585

22 Amouzou A, Hazel E, Shaw B, Miller NP, Tafesse M, Mekonnen Y, et al. Effects of the integrated community case management of childhood illness strategy on child mortality in Ethiopia: A cluster randomized trial. Am J Trop Med Hyg. 2016;94:596-604. Medline:26787148 doi:10.4269/ajtmh.15-0586

23 Shaw B, Amouzou A, Miller NP, Tsui AO, Bryce J, Tafesse M, et al. Determinants of Utilization of Health Extension Workers in the Context of Scale-Up of Integrated Community Case Management of Childhood Illnesses in Ethiopia. Am J Trop Med Hyg. 2015;93:636-47. Medline:26195461 doi:10.4269/ajtmh.14-0660

24 Phillips JF, Bawah AA, Binka FN. Accelerating reproductive and child health programme impact with community-based services: the Navrongo experiment in Ghana. Bull World Health Organ. 2006;84:949-55. Medline:17242830 doi:10.2471/BLT.06.030064

25 Nyonator FK, Jones TC, Miller RA, Phillips JF, Awoonor-Williams JK. Guiding the Ghana community-based health planning and services approach to scaling up with qualitative systems appraisal. Int Q Community Health Educ. 2004-2005;23:189-213. doi:10.2190/NGM3-FYDT-5827-ML1P

26 Marcil L, Afsana K, Perry HB. First steps in initiating an effective maternal, neonatal, and child health program in urban slums: the BRAC Manoshi Project's experience with community engagement, social mapping, and census taking in Bangladesh. J Urban Health. 2016;93:6-18. Medline:26830423 doi:10.1007/s11524-016-0026-0

27 Perry H, Davis T. The effectiveness of the census-based, impact-oriented (CBIO) approach in addressing global health goals. In: E. B, editor. Aid Effectiveness in Global Health. New York: Springer; 2015.

28 Black RE, Taylor CE, Arole S, Bang A, Bhutta ZA, Chowdhury AMR, et al. A comprehensive review of the evidence regarding the effectiveness of community-based primary health care in improving maternal, neonatal and child health: 8. conclusions and recommendations of an Expert Panel. J Glob Health. 2017;7:010908.

Acknowledgement: *originally published as: Paul A Freeman, Meike Schleiff, Emma Sacks, Bahie M Rassekh, Sundeep Gupta, Henry B Perry:Comprehensive review of the evidence regarding the effectiveness of Community–Based Primary Health Care in improving maternal, neonatal and child health:4. child health findings. Reprinted with permission from Edinburgh University Global Health Society under Creative Commons Attribution Licence (Journal of Global Health 2017; 010904).*

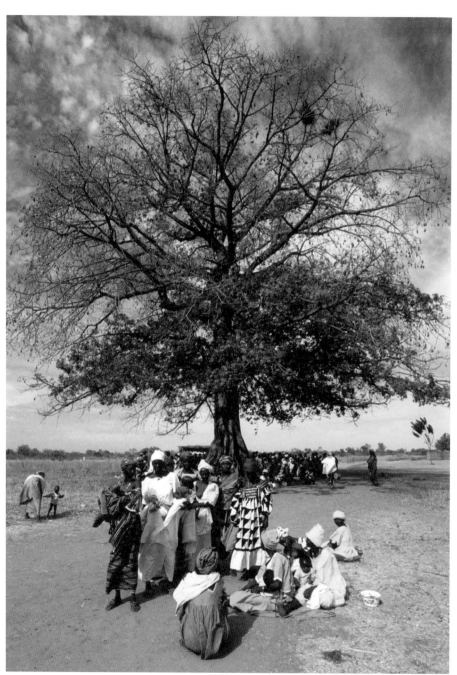

Photo credit: Dr Martin W. Weber, personal collection (used with permission).

Comprehensive review of the evidence regarding the effectiveness of community–based primary health care in improving maternal, neonatal and child health: 5. equity effects for neonates and children

**Meike Schleiff[1], Richard Kumapley[2], Paul A Freeman[3,4],
Sundeep Gupta[5], Bahie M Rassekh[6], Henry B Perry[1]**

[1] Department of International Health, Johns Hopkins Bloomberg School of Public Health, Baltimore, Maryland, USA
[2] UNICEF, New York, New York, USA
[3] Independent consultant, Seattle, Washington, USA
[4] Department of Global Health, University of Washington, Seattle, Washington, USA
[5] Medical epidemiologist, Lusaka, Zambia
[6] The World Bank, Washington, DC, USA

Background The degree to which investments in health programs improve the health of the most disadvantaged segments of the population—where utilization of health services and health status is often the worst—is a growing concern throughout the world. Therefore, questions about the degree to which community–based primary health care (CBPHC) can or actually does improve utilization of health services and the health status of the most disadvantaged children in a population is an important one.

Methods Using a database containing information about the assessment of 548 interventions, projects or programs (referred to collectively as projects) that used CBPHC to improve child health, we extracted evidence related to equity from a sub–set of 42 projects, identified through a multi–step process, that included an equity analysis. We organized our findings conceptually around a logical framework matrix.

Results Our analysis indicates that these CBPHC projects, all of which implemented child health interventions, achieved equitable effects. The vast majority (87%) of the 82 equity measurements carried out and reported for these 42 projects demonstrated "pro–equitable" or "equitable" effects, meaning that the project's equity indicator(s) improved to the same degree or more in the disadvantaged segments of the project population as in the more advantaged segments. Most (78%) of the all the measured equity effects were "pro–equitable," meaning that the equity criterion improved <u>more</u> in the most disadvantaged segment of the project population than in the other segments of the population.

Conclusions Based on the observation that CBPHC projects commonly provide services that are readily accessible to the entire project population and that even often reach down to all households, such projects are inherently likely to be more equitable than projects that strengthen services only at facilities, where utilization diminishes greatly with one's distance away. The decentralization of services and attention to and tracking of metrics across all phases of project implementation with attention to the underserved, as can be done in CBPHC projects, are important for reducing inequities in countries with a high burden of child mortality. Strengthening CBPHC is a necessary strategy for reducing inequities in child health and for achieving universal coverage of essential services for children.

Martin Luther King, Jr., in a speech in 1966 to the Medical Committee for Human Rights, proclaimed, *"Of all the forms of inequality, injustice in health care is the most shocking and inhumane"* [1]. Between countries and within countries, inequalities in health status are by and large considered inequitable because they can be greatly reduced or even eliminated through stronger health programs. In spite of marked improvements in health programming and health status around the world, inequities are not diminishing as much as many countries and stakeholders had hoped [2–4]. Particularly since the 1990s, measuring and working to reduce inequities — with a goal ultimately to reach zero — has been on the global health agenda from global and national policy–makers to major donors [3–6].

Issues of health inequities for maternal, neonatal and child health (MNCH) in low– and middle–income countries (LMICs) are being increasingly studied. Some progress is being made in a number of areas such as the use of insecticide–treated net (ITN) usage to prevent malaria, exclusive breastfeeding, and immunization coverage [7]. Further, approaches for reaching underserved populations are receiving increasing attention in order to achieve the Millennium Development Goals (MDGs) [4] and the newly established Sustainable Development Goals (SDGs) [8]. At the global level, a recent declaration [9] brought together national public health associations from around the world to focus and mobilize action for achieving health equity by building evidence, addressing the social determinants of health (SDH), and incorporating equity components into health policies. Nonetheless, a great deal of learning and work remains to be done in order to accelerate reductions in health inequities.

Recent evidence from tracking of the "Countdown to 2015" [7–12], when the MDGs were supposed to be achieved, shows that population coverage of key interventions provided by health services is improving for the poorest quintiles of national populations at a rate faster than that for the wealthiest quintiles. However, the poorest quintiles are still facing markedly lower levels of coverage than the wealthier quintiles in most Countdown countries (the 74 countries with 97% of the world's child and maternal deaths, ie, the greatest burden of maternal, neonatal and child mortality). Even though some measures of health inequities are slowly improving, substantial challenges remain for how to accelerate this progress [3,4]. The gaps are wider for interventions that require access to fixed health facilities or repeat contacts with a health provider (such as a skilled birth attendant) than for interventions that can be delivered through outreach strategies at the community level [5]. The countries that have made rapid progress in coverage are those that effectively reached the poorest families [5]. This is despite starting with great inequities. For example, in Cambodia and Sierra Leone in 2000 the richest had much higher coverage than the rest, but by 2014 this difference had disappeared [13].

The terminology around inequities, inequalities, and disparities has been the topic of debate over the past decades [14]. We will use the following interpretations of the terms in the context of this article. *Disparities* and *inequalities* (often used interchangeably) refer to differences among socially or geographically defined groups in health service utilization, in risk factors for unfavorable health outcomes, in levels of morbidity or mortality (collectively referred to here as health status) – essentially encompassing the entirety of epidemiological inquiry [14]. *Inequity*, however, "does not refer generically to all differences in health, but focuses specifically on the sub–set of differences that are 'avoidable, unfair, and unjust" [14]. In practice, studies of inequities in health often focus on the degree to which marginalized and disadvantaged groups within geographically defined populations have less access to health care resources and have lower utilization of health care services.

Such differences stem from characteristics such as educational level, income (or wealth), race, child's gender, geographic location, religion, or other characteristics of a social group that persistently produce social barriers that can lead to health outcomes that are different from those of other social groups. Beyond the semantics, Braveman argues that how we define and use these terms has important and relevant implications for policy and practice, and these definitions can determine the measures used to determine progress and even the flow of funding for different interventions [14]. Alternately, Taylor suggested a definition of equity as the, "distribution of benefits according to demonstrated need [health status] rather than on the basis of political or socioeconomic privilege" [15]. He focused on equity of the health status of populations rather than more proximal indicators of health system inputs or health service utilization.

From a public health perspective, it is important to examine the equity of both health program implementation and health outcomes among different socially and geographically defined sub–populations. Overall improvements in the health of a population can occur without every sub–group benefiting equally [7,16,17].

The equity effects of MNCH programs have undergone perhaps the greatest scrutiny of any global health program. One of the recent drivers for this scrutiny was the challenge of meeting the MDGs by 2015 and accelerating progress in countries that were lagging behind [11,12,18]. Analysts observed that, within many countries, inequities in child mortality were widening in spite of overall downward trends in child mortality [19].

Analyses have been conducted using Demographic and Health Survey (DHS) and Multiple Indicator Survey (MICS) data from MDG Countdown Countries regarding the population coverage of key maternal and child health interventions by income quintiles to assess equity in coverage [4,5]. Results showed trends toward increased equity in coverage of key interventions. Some of the most equitably implemented interventions are those that can fairly easily be implemented within communities, such as ITN utilization, promotion of exclusive breastfeeding (EBF), and community–based provision of immunizations [7,10,20,21]. At the same time, widening inequities were observed among different population sub–groups for interventions that require facility–based, higher–level personnel such as skilled birth attendants and treatment of serious childhood illness [22]. These interventions often require a more developed health system including education and support of skilled personnel, more advanced equipment, referral processes, and other support structures in order to be effective, and thus tend to be less evenly distributed among population groups [7,10].

While equity issues are often considered from a national or large–population perspective, they may exist at the local level as well. In one long–standing comprehensive health program in Haiti serving 148 000 people with a strong community–based service delivery system, the utilization of health facilities, the population coverage of key interventions, and the health outcomes of sub–groups of the program area differed markedly among those living in the more isolated mountain communities compared to those is nearer valley communities. This reality persisted despite great efforts being made to extend both primary health care services and access to CHWs equally throughout the program area [23].

This article makes two contributions to the equity literature. First, it consolidates for the first time the evidence regarding the equity effects of CBPHC programs on child health and organizes them around a logical framework.

Second, this article reviews the various dimensions of equity that child health programs need to consider, including wealth (or household assets), maternal education, child's sex, geographic location, and gender of the child's caregiver and identifies dimensions where limited analysis has been conducted.

METHODS

Data sources

We used a recently assembled database containing assessments of 548 studies, projects or programs (referred to collectively as projects) that used CBPHC (defined in the initial paper in this series [24]) to improve neonatal or child health (henceforth referred to as child health) and to document these improvements. In brief, CBPHC was considered to be one or more interventions carried out in the community outside of a health facility. The additional presence of one or more facility–based interventions did not disqualify the project from inclusion.

The database and its assembly have been described elsewhere in this series [10]. In short, peer–reviewed documents, reports and books assessing the impact of one or more CBPHC interventions on child health (coverage of a key child survival indicator, nutritional status, serious morbidity, or mortality) in LMIC settings, among children in a geographically defined population, were selected. Two independent data extraction reviews were carried out and followed by an independent consolidated summative review. Data from the latter review were transferred to electronic database.

From this database, we identified a sub–set of 42 projects that had carried out an equity analysis as part of their assessment using the process described in the following section.

Article review and inclusion process

Using the PRISMA guidelines for systematic reviews on health equity [25,26], we identified a sub–set of 138 articles in which equity was mentioned in one or more of the following fields in the CBPHC project database: 1) the title of the article, 2) the documentation of the process of the intervention, 3) part of the data analysis strategy, or 4) in the notes provided by the reviewers of the assessment for inclusion in the systematic review. We carefully reviewed this sub–set of equity–relevant assessments and excluded assessments in which equity was not actually analyzed across population subgroups. After this focusing phase, we were left with 43 projects to examine further.

Two of the authors (MS and RK) separately reviewed each of these 43 projects and extracted additional data on how equity was defined in each assessment, what data sources were utilized for assessment of equity effects, and what the outcome on equity actually was. The metrics from each project being assessed were stratified into log–frame categories (input, process, output, outcome, impact). One article was excluded from the analysis because it did not provide sufficient information on how equity was analyzed, leaving 42 articles in the final data set (**Figure 1**). Aside from the availability of adequate information on equity analysis in each article, the quality of the study was not assessed.

Criteria for equity analysis

In order to identify the diverse criteria utilized among the studies to analyze equity, we created open–text responses as we reviewed each assessment, and then categorized them into common themes as we identified commonalities among the identified categories. We summarize the categories below and provide examples for some of the less–common categories. In our literature review, we identified a USAID report [27] on incorporating equity into project designs for MNCH that offered guidance on identifying disadvantaged groups that should be considered in implementing equitable MNCH projects. The USAID report referred to these groups by the acronym PROGRESS (**P**lace of residence, **R**ace, **O**ccupation, **G**ender, **R**eligion, **E**ducation, and **S**ocioeconomic

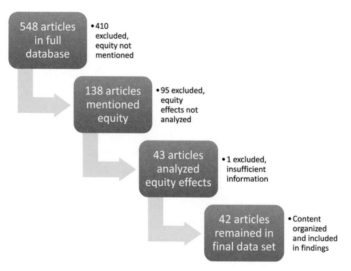

Figure 1. *Overview of sequence of article review and inclusion/exclusion criteria.*

Status) [28]. This typology provided guidance for the kinds of characteristics to look for and how to organize the findings from the reports we analyzed.

Categorization of equity outcomes

We created three categories of outcomes for the various equity indicators used by the assessments included in our analysis (pro–equitable, equitable, and inequitable, as defined in **Box 1**). We categorized indicators as pro–equitable if findings favored underserved populations and were statistically significant or, if tests of statistical significance were not carried out, the study authors described their results as having practical significance. Indicators with findings that were similar for underserved groups as for the other groups were categorized as equitable. Indicators with findings that showed unfavorable outcomes for underserved populations were categorized as inequitable.

These categories helped us to differentiate between several important equity outcomes –namely when disadvantaged sub–groups were benefitting less, equally, or more than other sub–groups. If disadvantaged groups were benefitting less, this was an inequitable outcome. When disadvantaged groups were benefitting equally, this was noted as a good sign, though not a fully optimal outcome since disadvantaged groups often need to make additional progress in order to overcome inequities.

Box 1. *Definitions*

> **Pro–equity effect:** when inputs, processes, and outcomes for disadvantaged groups improved more than for advantaged groups by the end of project implementation.
>
> **Equity effect:** when inputs, processes, and outcomes for disadvantaged groups improved to the same degree as advantaged groups by the end of project implementation.
>
> **Inequity effect:** when inputs, processes and outcomes for disadvantaged groups improve less than for advantaged groups by the end of project implementation.
>
> **Dimension of equity:** A characteristic — such as household income, level of maternal education, or whether a child lives in an urban or rural areas — that can be used to compare population groups through an equity lens and determine whether different sub–groups of the population receive different levels of services or achieve different outcomes.
>
> **Equity indicator:** An indicator of child health—such as rates of home visitation for newborns, for example — that was analyzed across a dimension of health equity.

Organization of identified metrics for health equity into a logical framework

Barros et al. [19] offer a framework for analysis of health equity from the standpoint of an individual person's experience with an illness, beginning with the socioeconomic context through exposures to disease, vulnerability to succumbing to disease, and the outcomes and consequences of illness. While this approach helped us think through the various ways that equity can influence child health work, we opted to organize the indicators of health equity used by the assessments included in our analysis by utilizing a different framework of analysis from the standpoint of project implementation: beginning with inputs and processes, and then moving to outputs, outcomes, and impacts [29] to track at what point in project implementation equity dimensions were assessed. This made it possible to identify gaps and opportunities from a project planning and implementation perspective. **Figure 2** below provides a graphic representation of the conceptual flow of this log–frame matrix from one phase to another.

We created a matrix for each phase of the logical framework and, for each of the included indicators, tabulated the equity effects of each project. For each cell of the matrix, we described the content of the project and drew conclusions from the available evidence.

Each assessment was further analyzed to determine the criteria used to define equity, the type of data used to assess equity, and the scope of the assessment as well as the types of indicators measured in the assessment. The definition of equity was not pre–determined, and the definitions of equity used in the assessments were categorized after the list of equity indicators used in the projects had been reviewed. This was done to avoid missing any relevant equity indicators that might not have fit into a pre–determined definition of equity.

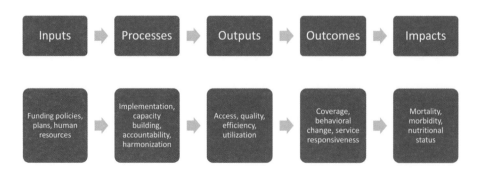

Figure 2. *Generalized log frame for health projects.*

The type of data used to assess equity was defined as primary or secondary. The term primary data refers to data collected by the project, while the term secondary data refers to data which were gathered by another entity. Secondary data included those obtained from DHS and MICS data sets. Finally, each indicator was further classified as to whether it was referring to a project input, process, output, outcome or impact.

RESULTS

Location of included projects

Table 1. *Geographical location of reports containing equity analyses*

GEOGRAPHICAL REGION	NUMBER OF STUDIES
Africa	19
Southeast Asia	14
Americas	8
Western Pacific	1
Total	42

The assessments included in our analysis were for projects from various regions of the world (**Table 1**). One of the studies included data from 28 African countries, and another had data from four African countries. All other studies focused on one country or a smaller sub–population within that country as shown in **Table 1**.

Kinds of data used in the assessments

The data utilized in 37 of the 42 projects including equity analyses collected specifically by the project within the project's geographic area. However, five analyses exclusively utilized data from DHS and MICS surveys, and two utilized both project–level data collected for assessment of the project and also publicly available national data.

Criteria through which equity effects were assessed

Across the 42 projects included in our analysis, 82 equity indicators — for example coverage of prenatal home visits analyzed across household income categories (Callaghan–Koru, 2013; reference [S15] in **Online Supplementary Document**) — were identified. Equity was measured by comparing changes in health program characteristics or health status over time for more disadvantaged groups with changes in the identical indicators for more advantaged groups. **Table 2** summarizes the criteria by which disadvantaged groups were distinguished from more advantaged groups.

We grouped several equity indicators under a category we refer to as socio-economic status (SES). These included income categories, maternal education, and household characteristics. By far, the most common indicator for assessing

Table 2. *Equity indicators used in the assessments included in the analysis*

EQUITY CRITERION	NUMBER OF ASSESS- MENTS IN WHICH THE INDICATOR WAS USED*	COMPARABLE USAID PROG- RESS INDICA- TORS
Socioeconomic status (SES):		
Household income categories	45	Wealth
Household assets (production, other assets such as savings)	5	Wealth
Maternal education	9	Gender
Social standing (ethnicity, caste, religion, parent marital status)	8	Ethnicity
Parent occupation	1	Wealth
Other:		
Geographic location of residence (urban vs rural)	24	Geography
Child's sex	3	Gender
Nutritional status	4	Wealth
Maternal age	2	Age
Country–level Human Development Index (HDI)	1	Wealth

*The column total is 82 since many of the assessments in our review included more than one equity indicator.

equity was a measure of wealth, often based on household income, household assets, household size, or maternal earnings. Other SES equity indicators included in the analysis were agricultural production by heads of household and specific assets present in the household such as a working toilet, running water, or a refuse collection system. Other SES criteria included the ethnic group of the family, religion, marital status of child's parents, occupation of the parents, and demographic characteristics such as maternal age. These equity indicators aligned well with those identified by the USAID PROGRESS report (shown in the right–hand column of **Table 2**); the only PROGRESS category that was not identified in our analysis was religion [27].

Assessments of equity of inputs

After careful analysis and discussion among co–authors and colleagues, we determined that no projects that we included in our data set explicitly analyzed or reported inputs from an equity perspective. The dearth of input–related efforts in project design, implementation, and evaluation is concerning and is noted as an area where further work is needed.

Assessments of equity of processes

A number of the assessments included in our review measured process indicators through an equity lens, as shown in **Table 3** (references in Tables 3–6, are prefixed with an S and appear in **Online Supplementary Document**).

Table 3. *Assessments of equity effects of CBPHC projects using process indicators**

PROCESS INDICATOR	EQUITY CRITERION	OUTCOME	REFERENCE
Postnatal home visit	Household income	Equitable	Callaghan–Koru 2013 [S15]
Home visit during pregnancy	Household income	Equitable	Callaghan–Koru 2013 [S15]
Azythromycin distribution to entire communities for trachoma	Household assets	Pro–equitable	Cumberland 2008 [S19]
CHW visit to caregivers within the past year	Urban vs rural	Pro–equitable	Litrell 2013 [S25]
Caregivers report of CHWs working in community	Urban vs rural	Pro–equitable	Litrell 2013 [S25]
Prenatal home visit	Household income	Pro–equitable	Baqui 2008 [S8]
Number of home visits	Urban vs rural	Pro–equitable	Perry 2006 [S35]
Antenatal home visit	Household income	Pro–equitable	Baqui 2008 [S8]
At least one home visit during pregnancy	Household income	Pro–equitable	Callaghan–Koru 2013 [S15]
Two or more home visits during pregnancy	Household income	Pro–equitable	Callaghan–Koru 2013 [S15]
Home visits to support breast-feeding	Household income, maternal education	Pro–equitable	Coutinho 2005 [S17]
Child ill and CHW called to come to the home	Household income	Pro–equitable	Siekmans 2013 [S38]
At least one ANC visit in home	Household income	Pro–equitable	Nonyane 2015 [S32]

*References which are prefixed with an S appear in Appendix S1 of the **online supplementary document**.

Two–thirds (10/13) of the measurements of equity involving process indicators concerned whether the household had received a home visit from a health worker or had contact with the health system. Eleven out of 13 of the measurements yielded a pro–equitable result, and the remaining two yielded an equitable result. Thus, for the process indicators in the assessments selected for analysis, equity had been achieved in all cases and a pro–equity result is observed in almost all. The findings for this portion of the log frame consistently support the equitable nature of home visiting practices, a central feature of many CBPHC projects, as also discussed in the in this supplement that directly address the effectiveness of CBPHC in improving MNCH [30–32]. Many of these home visits either implicitly or explicitly included promotion and support of breastfeeding, which has also been noted in the literature as an intervention that can be supported equitably through community–based approaches with multiple benefits to MNCH.

Assessments of equity of outputs

The assessments of equity using output indicators are listed in **Table 4**. Two–thirds (4/6) of the six equity assessments using output indicators among the

Table 4. *Assessments of equity effects of CBPHC projects using output indicators**

OUTPUT INDICATOR	EQUITY CRITERION	OUTCOME	REFERENCE
Food hygiene score in relation to cleanliness score	Household income	Inequitable	Ahmed 1993 [S1]
Food hygiene score in relation to diarrhea prevalence	Maternal education, nutritional status	Inequitable	Ahmed 1993 [S1]
Utilization of ambulatory care facility	Urban vs rural	Pro–equitable	Perry 2006 [S35]
Number of hospital admissions	Urban vs rural	Pro–equitable	Perry 2006 [S35]
Child with fever treated within 24 h	Household income	Pro–equitable	Siekmans 2013 [S38]
Essential newborn practices performed	Household income	Pro–equitable	Baqui 2008 [S8]

*References which are prefixed with an S appear in Appendix S1 of the **online supplementary document**.

projects selected for our analysis concerned the utilization of specific services or the expected immediate output of an intervention. Half (3/6) of these equity assessments used household income as the equity criterion. The number of assessments is too small to make major generalizations from, but the indicators demonstrating a pro–equity effect in the output category focus on access to health services (either in a facility or in the home). Indicators that demonstrated an inequitable effect were both from the same study and related to the hygienic practices across several equity dimensions.

Assessments of equity of outcomes

Table 5 below lists the equity assessments carried out using outcome indicators. Many relate to knowledge and behavior change related to breastfeeding or to the population coverage level of an intervention. Of the 35 measurement carried out, only 14% (5/35) yielded an inequitable result; 11% (4/35) yielded an equitable result, and the rest (74%) yielded a pro–equitable result. Inequitable indicators included several interventions requiring significant equipment or knowledge such as vaccine coverage and antenatal and delivery care. Some indicators — such as ITN coverage, availability, and use — showed mixed results across different studies, with some having equitable results across household income categories or urban and rural settings and others not. Equitable and pro–equitable programs commonly focused on equitable behaviors such as breastfeeding and newborn and child health practices that can be implemented in the home without complex or expensive supplies or knowledge.

Assessments of equity of health impact

Finally, **Table 6** lists the assessments of health equity that were carried out for health impact–related indicators (nutritional status, morbidity or mortality). Of the 28 projects that included an equity assessment of health impact, 20 were

Table 5. *Assessments of equity effects of CBPHC projects using outcome indicators**

Outcome indicator	Equity criterion	Outcome	Reference
Understanding of overall cleanliness	Maternal education	Inequitable	Ahmed 1993 [S1]
Coverage of antenatal and delivery care	Household income	Inequitable	Bryce 2008 [S14]
EPI immunization coverage	Household income	Inequitable	Webster 2005 [S42]
ITN coverage	Household income	Inequitable	Webster 2005 [S42]
Coverage of any type of bed net (ITN or other)	Household income	Inequitable	Webster 2005 [S42]
Health service coverage	Child's sex	Equitable	Bryce 2008 [S14]
Nothing applied to umbilical cord by mother after birth	Household income	Equitable	Nonyane 2015 [S32]
Child with diarrhea treated with ORS or zinc	Household income	Equitable	Littrell 2013 [S25]
Awareness of support group in community	Household income	Equitable	Callaghan–Koru 2013 [S15]
Exclusive breastfeeding	Urban vs rural	Pro–equitable	Crookston 2000 [S18]
Exclusive breastfeeding from birth to 6m	Household income	Pro–equitable	Coutinho 2005 [S17]
Breastfeeding initiation within first hour of life	Urban vs rural	Pro–equitable	Crookston 2000 [S17]
Breastfeeding initiation within first hour of life	Household income	Pro–equitable	Nonyane 2015 [S32]
Knowledge of family planning methods	Urban vs rural	Pro–equitable	Debpuur 2002 [S20]
Knowledge and use of family planning	Maternal education, social standing	Pro–equitable	Awooner–Williams 2004 [S5]
Recognition of at least 3 danger signs in newborns	Household income	Pro–equitable	Nonyane 2015 [S32]
Child with fever treated with artemether–lumefantrine within 48 hours	Household income	Pro–equitable	Siekmans 2013 [S38]
Acute respiratory infection treatment rate	Household income	Pro–equitable	Mercer 2004 [S28]
Any bed net available	Household income	Pro–equitable	Skarbinski 2007 [S39]
Measles vaccination rate	Household income	Pro–equitable	Mercer 2004 [S28]
Immunization coverage	Household income	Pro–equitable	Bawah 2006 [S10]
ITN in home	Household income	Pro–equitable	Skarbinski 2007 [S39]
ITN coverage	Urban vs rural	Pro–equitable	Grabowsky 2005 [S23]
ITN coverage	Household income	Pro–equitable	Grabowsky 2005 [S23]
ITN coverage	Household income	Pro–equitable	Noor 2007 [S33]
Immediate drying	Household income	Pro–equitable	Nonyane 2015 [S32]
Postnatal care coverage	Maternal education, household income, social standing, household assets	Pro–equitable	Awooner–Williams 2004 [S5]
Children sleeping under ITNs	Household income	Pro–equitable	Noor 2007 [S33]
Attended delivery	Maternal education, household income, social standing, household assets	Pro–equitable	Awooner–Williams 2004 [S5]
Antenatal care	Maternal education, household income, social standing, household assets	Pro–equitable	Awooner–Williams 2004 [S5]
Antenatal care coverage	Household income	Pro–equitable	Baqui 2008 [S8]

*References which are prefixed with an S appear in Appendix S1 of the **online supplementary document**.

Table 6. *Assessments of equity of CBPHC projects using impact indicators**

IMPACT INDICATOR	EQUITY CRITERION	OUTCOME	REFERENCE
Neonatal morality rate	Household income	Inequitable	Razzaque 2007 [S36]
Under–5 mortality rate	Urban vs rural	Inequitable	Bryce 2008 [S14]
Under–5 mortality rate	Household income	Inequitable	Razzaque 2007 [S36]
Child (age 6–59 months) mortality rate	Social standing, child's sex	Inequitable	Bishai 2005 [S12]
Tetanus neonatorum mortality rate	Urban vs rural	Equitable	Newell 1966 [S31]
Diarrhea prevalence in children 0–36 months of age	Urban vs rural	Pro–equitable	Barreto 2007 [S9]
Diarrhea prevalence in children 0–18 months of age	Nutritional status	Pro–equitable	Ahmed 1993 [S1]
Diarrhea prevalence in children 0–36 months of age	Urban vs rural	Pro–equitable	Barreto 2007 [S9]
Undernutrition prevalence	Nutritional status	Pro–equitable	Mustaphi 2005 [S30]
Child nutrition status (qualitative data)	Nutritional status	Pro–equitable	McNelly 1998 [S29]
Perinatal mortality rate	Urban vs rural	Pro–equitable	Bang 2005 [S7]
Perinatal mortality rate	Urban vs rural	Pro–equitable	Bang 1999 [S6]
Neonatal mortality rate	Urban vs rural	Pro–equitable	ASHA–India 2008 [S4]
Neonatal mortality rate	Urban vs rural	Pro–equitable	Bang 1999 [S6]
Infant mortality rate	Maternal education, child's sex	Pro–equitable	Fegan 2007 [S21]
Infant mortality rate	Urban vs rural	Pro–equitable	Asha–India 2008 [S4]
Infant mortality rate	Social standing, parental occupation	Pro–equitable	Bang 1999 [S6]
Infant mortality rate	Household income	Pro–equitable	Bhuiya 2002 [S11]
Infant mortality rate	Household assets, maternal education	Pro–equitable	Bang 2005 [S7]
Infant mortality rate	Human development index	Pro–equitable	Aquino 2009 [S2]
Infant mortality rate	Household income	Pro–equitable	Mercer 2004 [S28]
Infant, 1–4 years, and under–5 mortality rates	Household income	Pro–equitable	Mercer 2004 [S28]
Under–5 mortality rate	Household income	Pro–equitable	Sepulveda 2006 [S37]
Under–5 mortality rate	Urban vs rural, household income	Pro–equitable	Asha–India 2008 [S4]
Under–5 mortality rate	Urban vs rural	Pro–equitable	Perry 2006 [S35]
Under–5 mortality rate	Household income	Pro–equitable	Bryce 2008 [S14]
Under–5 mortality rate	Urban vs rural	Pro–equitable	Asha–India 2008 [S4]

*References which are prefixed with an S appear in Appendix S1 of the **online supplementary document**.

based on a measure of mortality; four were based on a measure of morbidity and four on a measure of nutritional status. Overall, 23 of the 28 assessments demonstrated pro–equitable results and one yielded an equitable result. Only four of the 28 yielded an inequitable result.

Overall summary of equity effects using household wealth as the equity criterion

We have summarized all the findings reported above in which household income was the equity criterion (**Table 7**). Overall, 75% (33/44) of these effects were pro–equitable outcome, 9% were equitable outcomes, and only 16% (7/44) yielded an inequitable effect.

Overall summary of all equity effects

Finally, we have summarized equity effects in **Table 8**. Overall, 78% (64/82) of the equity assessments carried out yielded a pro–equitable outcome; 9% (7/82) yielded an equitable outcomes, and only 13% (11/82) yielded an inequitable outcome.

While in–depth analysis of the impact of packages of interventions was not the focus of this paper (another paper in this series [33] addresses this strategy in general – not limited to equity), we reviewed which projects constituted a single intervention vs a package of interventions. Of the 42 projects, 11 (26%) included a single intervention while eight (19%) included 2 interventions,

Table 7. *Summary of assessments of equity using socio–economic status or household wealth quintile as the equity criterion*

TYPE OF INDICATOR	EFFECT ON EQUITY			
	Inequitable	Equitable	Pro–equitable	Total
Input	0	0	0	0
Process	0	2	7	9
Output	1	0	2	3
Outcome	4	2	18	24
Impact	2	0	6	8
Total	7	4	33	44

Table 8. *Summary of all assessments of equity*

TYPE OF INDICATOR	EFFECT ON EQUITY			
	Inequitable	Equitable	Pro–equitable	Total
Input	0	0	0	0
Process	0	2	11	13
Output	2	0	4	6
Outcome	5	4	26	35
Impact	4	1	23	28
Total	11	7	64	82

and 23 (55%) of projects had a package of three or more services. We could not identify any clear patterns between the number of interventions and how equitable the findings were; the only clear pattern was that, in general, all interventions and equity dimensions within any particularly project tended to be the same in terms of equity outcomes (eg, all of the findings for Ahmed 1993 were inequitable).

Of the 42 projects that conducted an equity analysis, we also reviewed which ones analyzed more one or more dimensions of equity. 27 (64%) included an analysis for only one dimension of equity while nine (21%) included two dimensions of equity, and only six (14%) included three or more dimensions of equity. We also did not identify any obvious patterns among the small groups of projects in each of these categories. Household income as part of SES was by far the most common dimension of equity, and was utilized across all of these categories followed closely by comparing urban vs rural populations. The projects with inequitable findings included a number of SES analyses and also child gender and an urban vs rural comparison.

DISCUSSION

We have carried out an equity analysis of the projects in our review that contained evidence regarding the equity effects of CBPHC in improving child health. Out of the 546 assessments related to child health in our data set, 42 measured equity effects. Of the 82 measurements of equity effects in these 42 projects, 87% of these measurements indicated that the equity effect was either equitable (in which the disadvantage group benefitted to the same degree as the more advantaged group) or pro–equitable (in which the disadvantaged group benefitted more). Of the 42 articles in our review, 15 of them (36%) measured two or more equity dimensions and 31 articles (74%) measured equity across two or more interventions. These findings provide strong evidence of the capacity of CPBHC to reduce inequities in the delivery of child health services and in child health outcomes. Thus, these findings are consistent with the assertion that CBPHC has the potential to reduce inequities in child health in low–income settings where health facilities alone would be highly unlikely to reduce existing inequities since, in fact, it is well–known that health facility utilization in low–income settings is highly inequitable, as explained further below.

The counter–argument to this assertion is that expansion of the number of facilities and improvements in facility–based care will eventually reduce inequities in child health. This may be possible in the very long term, but there is no evidence at present that we are aware of demonstrating that expanding or improving facility–based services as an isolated strategy reduces inequities in the delivery of child health services or in child health status. For the near term, resources will continue to be highly constrained in low–income countries and major geographic [34], social and financial barriers will continue to exist in accessing facility–based care. Therefore, our findings indicate that strong expansion of CBPHC will be required to reduce inequities in child health.

A case example from Brazil of equity effects of CBPHC on improving child health (an article selected from database) serves as an example of the potential pro–equity effects of combining community–based approaches with political will and investment, a national strategy, and a long-term commitment).

Aquino et al., 2008 (reference [S12] in **Online Supplementary Document**) analyzed the effects of expanding Brazil's Family Health Program (FHP) coverage on infant mortality. They identified that the effect of the FHP program was greatest in terms of decreasing infant mortality in municipalities where infant mortality was highest and the human development index was lowest at the beginning of the study period. The FHP program used a family–centered approach to provide a range of services at the community level, including promotion of breastfeeding, prenatal care, immunizations, and management of diarrhea. The team of health workers, in addition to physicians and nurses as well as oral health professionals, includes CHWs (called Community Health Agents) who visited every home on a monthly basis. This national program has brought Brazil global recognition for its efforts to reduce health inequities for the general population and for children in particular (including inequities of childhood nutritional status). A high level of political will has been necessary in order to implement the scale and depth of this program at the national level.

Explaining the pro–equity effects of community–based primary health care

Most CBPHC projects are designed to reach every household with health education and information about how to access outreach services (if not to actually provide services including curative care), and outreach services are generally distributed more evenly throughout target populations than facility–based services [35]. Meanwhile, some countries, such as Peru, where great investment in health facilities has taken place — including expansion of community health centers — these efforts have resulted in only very small improvements on equitable utilization of health facilities [36].

Research on the equity of facility utilization in low–income settings is limited; more evidence is available for high–income settings in the Americas, Europe, and Asia. In LMIC settings, health facilities tend to be few and far between, often expensive from the perspective of the poor, and lacking high quality of care, including provision of care that is seen by certain sub–groups as disrespectful [36–38]. Factors such as education level, income, and urban and rural residence play key roles in determining whether someone is more or less likely to seek care at a health facility [36,37]. Thus, the effort and resources that patients and their families have to expend to reach a health facility and the uncertain return on that family's investment contributes to low utilization of facility–based services.

The challenge of providing interventions that are often only available in health facilities – or require infrastructure and skills difficult to deploy in communities outside of facilities — is significant as well. A growing literature, including but also going beyond the database used in this study, points to inequitable usage of health facilities in terms of the SES and urban/rural characteristics of users [23,34,39].

The need for alternative approaches beyond health facilities to achieve equity in and in fact universal coverage for child health are the following: (i) there is an exponential decline in the utilization of health facilities with increasing distance to the health facility (particularly more than 5 km or 1 hour walk away) [35], and (ii) there is a need for available and affordable public transportation in order to reach health facilities, which is often absent [33,39]. What is lacking from the literature are in–depth assessments of equity of health care utilization in terms of distance from a health facility and the effect of distance from health facilities on health status, taking into account also whether community–based care is available to those further away from those facilities.

Strong community–based programs can encourage facility utilization across income strata as can vouchers provided at the community level for specific services, such as antenatal care, to reduce resource barriers to seeking care [40]. The available evidence suggests that CBPHC approaches that reach all households can be more equitable than solely facility–based approaches in terms of coverage of a number of key primary health care services, particularly for vulnerable populations and those who live further away from facilities, who are also usually more disadvantaged in terms of SES [20,41–43].

There are several assessments that directly compare the degree to which CB-PHC approaches as opposed to other approaches improve the health of the poorest segment of the project population compared to hat of the better off segment. It makes sense that home–centered, low–resource interventions like breastfeeding promotion and distribution of ITNs would be able to achieve high levels of equity through community–based approaches that often include direct contact with all households [7]. In addition, some of the most promising strategies to improve health equity focus on strengthening community outreach, using CHWs and other lay workers, along with market–driven options such as minimizing or removing user fees and engaging the private sector [3,44,45].

Approaches that make it possible for health workers to reach all households – or at least to reach outreach points that are relatively evenly distributed throughout the project population and close to homes – are inherently more likely to achieve favorable equity effects than facility–based approaches. However, a number of other equity–relevant factors including education, child's sex, ethnicity [46], and urban vs rural contexts [47] cannot be overlooked even within such a strong outreach approach [48]. Health programs in high–mortality, resource–constrained settings lack the capacity to build and operate facilities within easy reach of all who could need to use them – particularly in low–density rural areas. Thus, the decentralization of services and utilization of innovative and proven strategies to support the coverage, quality, and sustainability of those services is essential for achieving health equity.

While the focus of this review is on low–income countries, inequities are also prevalent in higher–income countries as well. Even where more resources are available to address such issues, political will is needed to direct those resources in ways that decrease inequities. An example of progress and success in the arena of health equity is Japan's national policies to provide equitable educational opportunities as well as access to health services without financial barriers [49]. Globally, but particularly in low–income countries, much work remains to be done to make this kind of progress a reality for all populations. In addition to our public health–specific tools and approaches, more comprehensive community development and empowerment frameworks, such as the CHOICE (Capacity–building, Human rights, Organizational sustainability, Institutional accountability, Contribution, and Enabling environment) framework [50], can help to frame issues of health equity and provide additional entry points for understanding and addressing them. As Victora et al. note [51], just using the data available and recognizing patterns in inequities is not enough; political will and deliberate design and attention to the causes of inequities in programs for child health are necessary to achieve substantial decreases in child mortality among the most disadvantaged sub–populations where the mortality rates are the greatest.

Community–based approaches can reach those furthest from health facilities and can rapidly expand population coverage of key interventions, so these findings are not surprising. These findings stand in stark contrast to the commonly observed finding that utilization of primary health care facilities is inequitable because those in the lower income quintiles are less likely to obtain services there [52,53]. To our knowledge, this is the first comprehensive review in the peer–reviewed literature summarizing the equity effects of CBPHC in improving child health.

Limitations of our study

This study has several limitations that we want to make explicit. First, we have not further disaggregated the articles based on how strong the equity effect is. Second, some of the 42 assessments qualifying for our analysis are efficacy studies conducted within community settings in which ideal conditions were present for project implementation. Therefore, we must be careful about generalizing these findings to everyday practice settings. But, that said, it still remains true that strong pro–equity effects are achievable through CBPHC. An analysis of the quality of the data included in the 42 assessments included in our review was beyond the scope of this article. Finally, although a thorough search has been conducted that covers articles published over the past six decades through the end of 2015, we know that there are likely to be more recent articles published since that time that are relevant to this analysis.

We have worked to be clear in our language, conservative in our claims, and yet optimistic about the role of community–based approaches to continue to help bolster health equity for children in disadvantaged populations around the world.

CONCLUSIONS

Based on the finding that the services provided by CBPHC projects generally reach most or all households and are readily accessible throughout the project population, CBPHC projects are inherently more likely to achieve pro–equity effects than projects that strengthen services only at facilities. The decentralization of service provision and management and the utilization of community–level workers are important for reducing inequities in national programs of countries where the risk of child mortality is high. Equity assessments need to become a standard feature of MNCH programming.

Acknowledgments: We are grateful to Jennifer Winestock Luna for her review of an earlier draft of this manuscript. We are grateful to the following organizations that provided small grants to cover the expenses of this review: UNICEF, the World Bank, the Department of Child and Adolescent Health and Development of the World Health Organization, the CORE Group (Collaboration and Resources for Child Health)/USAID, Future Generations, and the Gates Foundation. We are also grateful to the American Public Health Association and particularly its International Health Section staff, which administered some of these funds. We thank Future Generations for providing office space, administrative support, and salary support to Dr Perry during the initial phase of the review. The World Bank made it possible for one of its consultants, Dr Bahie Rassekh, to participate as a member of the Study Team.

Funding: *The following organizations provided funds that were used to conduct the work described in this article: The World Health Organization, UNICEF, the World Bank, the United States Agency for International Development, and the Gates Foundation. The organizations that provided financial support had no role in the execution of the review.*

Authorship declaration: *MS wrote the first draft. RK and MS conducted the primary analysis of the data. All of the authors participated in the revision of earlier drafts and approved the final draft.*

Conflict of interest: *All authors have completed the Unified Competing Interest Form at www.icmje.org/coi_disclosure.pdf (available upon request from the corresponding author), and declare no conflict of interest.*

References

1 Moore A. Tracking Down Martin Luther King, Jr.'s Words on Health Care. 2013. Available: http://www.huffingtonpost.com/amanda-moore/martin-luther-king-health-care_b_2506393.html. Accessed: 20 March 2017.

2 Barros AJ, Victora CG. Measuring Coverage in MNCH: determining and interpreting inequalities in coverage of maternal, newborn, and child health interventions. PLoS Med. 2013;10:e1001390. Medline:23667332 doi:10.1371/journal.pmed.1001390

3 McCollum R, Gomez W, Theobald S, Taegtmeyer M. How equitable are community health worker programmes and which programme features influence equity of community health workers services? A systematic review. BMC Public Health. 2016;16:419. Medline:27207151 doi:10.1186/s12889-016-3043-8

4 Requejo J, Victora C, Bryce J. A Decade of Tracking Progress for Maternal, Newborn, and Child Survival: The 2015 Report. Baltimore, MD: Johns Hopkins University, 2015.

5 Barros AJ, Ronsmans C, Axelson H, Loaiza E, Bertoldi AD, Franca GV, et al. Equity in maternal, newborn, and child health interventions in Countdown to 2015: a retrospective review of survey data from 54 countries. Lancet. 2012;379:1225-33. Medline:22464386 doi:10.1016/S0140-6736(12)60113-5

6 Requejo JH, Bryce J, Barros AJ, Berman P, Bhutta Z, Chopra M, et al. Countdown to 2015 and beyond: fulfilling the health agenda for women and children. Lancet. 2015;385:466-76. Medline:24990815 doi:10.1016/S0140-6736(14)60925-9

7 Barros AJ, Ronsmans C, Axelson H, Loaiza E, Bertoldi A. Equity in Maternal, Newborn, and Child Health Interventions in Countdown to 2015: A Retrospective Review of Survey Data from 54 Countries. Lancet. 2012;379:1225-33. Medline:22464386 doi:10.1016/S0140-6736(12)60113-5

8 Victora CG, Requejo JH, Barros AJ, Berman P, Bhutta Z, Boerma T, et al. Countdown to 2015: a decade of tracking progress for maternal, newborn, and child survival. Lancet. 2016;387:2049-59. Medline:26477328 doi:10.1016/S0140-6736(15)00519-X

9 World Federation of Public Health Associations. The Addis Ababa Declaration on Global Health Equity: A Call To Action. 2012. Available: http://www.wfpha.org/tl_files/doc/about/Addis_Declaration.pdf. Accessed: 20 March 2017.

10   Countdown 2008 Equity Analysis Group, Boerma JT, Bryce J, Kinfu Y, Axelson H, Victora CG. Mind The Gap: equity and trends in coverage of maternal, newborn, and child health services in 54 Countdown Countries. Lancet. 2008;371:1259-67. Medline:18406860 doi:10.1016/S0140-6736(08)60560-7

11   Victora CG, Barros A, Axelson H, Bhutta J, Chopra M, Franca G, et al. How changes in coverage affect equity in maternal and child health interventions in 35 Countdown to 2015 countries: an analysis of national surveys. Lancet. 2012;380:1149-56. Medline:22999433 doi:10.1016/S0140-6736(12)61427-5

12   Barros AJ, Ronsmans C, Axelson H, Loaiza E, Bertoldi AD, França GV, et al. Equity in maternal, newborn, and child health interventions in Countdown to 2015: a retrospective review of survey data from 54 countries. Lancet. 2012;379:1225-33. Medline:22464386 doi:10.1016/S0140-6736(12)60113-5

13   UNICEF, World Health Organization. A Decade of Tracking Progress for Maternal, Newborn and Child Survival: The 2015 Report. 2015. Available: http://www.countdown2015mnch.org/documents/2015Report/Countdown_to_2015_final_report.pdf. Accessed: 20 March 2017.

14   Braveman P. Health disparities and health equity: concepts and measurement. Annu Rev Public Health. 2006;27:167-94. Medline:16533114 doi:10.1146/annurev.publhealth.27.021405.102103

15   Taylor CE. Surveillance for equity in primary health care: policy implications from international experience. Int J Epidemiol. 1992;21:1043-9. Medline:1483808 doi:10.1093/ije/21.6.1043

16   World Health Organization. Closing the Gap in a Generation: Health Equity Through Action on the Social Determinants of Health. Geneva: World Health Organization; 2008.

17   Hofman K, Blomstedt Y, Addei S, Kalage R, Maredza M, Sankoh O, et al. Addressing research capacity for health equity and the social determinants of health in three African countries: the INTREC Programme. Glob Health Action. 2013;6:19668. doi:10.3402/gha.v6i0.19668

18   Marmot M, Bell R. Social inequalities in health: a proper concern for epidemiology. Ann Epidemiol. 2016;26:238-40. Medline:27084546 doi:10.1016/j.annepidem.2016.02.003

19   Barros F, Victora C, Scherpbier R, Gwatkin D. Health and Nutrition of Children: Equity and Social Determinants. In: Blas E, Kurup AS, editors. Equity, Social Determinants, and Public Health Programmes. Geneva: World Health Organization; 2010.

20   Gilmour S, Shibuya K. Simple steps to equity in child survival. BMC Med. 2013;11:261. Medline:24344755 doi:10.1186/1741-7015-11-261

21   Afsana K, Haque MR, Sobhan S, Shahin SA. BRAC's Experience in scaling-up MNP in Bangladesh. Asia Pac J Clin Nutr. 2014;23:377-84. Medline:25164447

22   World Health Organization. Ending Preventable Child Deaths from Pneumonia and Diarrhea by 2025: The Integrated Global Action Plan for Pneumonia and Diarrhea (GAPPD). Geneva: World Health Organization; 2013.

23   Perry HB, King-Schultz L, Aftab A, Bryant J. Health equity issues at the local level: socio-geography, access, and health outcomes in the service area of the Hôpital Albert Schweitzer-Haiti. Int J Equity Health. 2007;6:7. Medline:17678540 doi:10.1186/1475-9276-6-7

24 Perry H, Rassekh B, Gupta S, Wilhelm J, Freeman P. A comprehensive review of the evidence regarding the effectiveness of community-based primary health care in improving maternal, neonatal and child health: 1. rationale, methods and database description. J Glob Health. 2017;7:010901.

25 Welch V, Tugwell P, Petticrew M, de Montigny J, Ueffing E, Kristjansson B, et al. How effects on health equity are assessed in systematic reviews of interventions. Cochrane Database Syst Rev. 2010;MR000028. Medline:21154402

26 Welch V, Petticrew M, Tugwell P, Moher D, O'Neill J, Waters E, et al. PRISMA-Equity 2012 extension: reporting guidelines for systematic reviews with a focus on health equity. PLoS Med. 2012;9:e1001333. Medline:23222917 doi:10.1371/journal.pmed.1001333

27 Winestock-Luna J, Victora C. Considerations for Incorporating Health Equity into Project Designs: A Guide for Community-Oriented Maternal, Neonatal, and Child Health Projects. Washington, DC: USAID, 2011.

28 Gwatkin DR. 10 Best resources on...health equity. Health Policy Plan. 2007;22:348-51. Medline:17698890 doi:10.1093/heapol/czm028

29 Bryce J, Victora CG, Boerma T, Peters DH, Black RE. Evaluating the scale-up for maternal and child survival: a common framework. Int Health. 2011;3:139-46. Medline:24038362 doi:10.1016/j.inhe.2011.04.003

30 Jennings MC, Pradhan S, Schleiff M, Sacks E, Freeman P, Gupta S. A comprehensive review of the evidence regarding the effectiveness of Community-based Primary Health Care in improving maternal, neonatal, and child health: 2.Maternal health Findings. J Glob Health. 2017;7:010902.

31 Sacks E, Freeman P, Jennings MC, Rassekh B, Gupta S, Perry H. A comprehensive review of the evidence regarding the effectiveness of Community-based Primary Health Care in improving maternal, neonatal, and child health: 3. neonatal health findings. J Glob Health. 2017;7:010903.

32 Freeman P, Schleiff M, Sacks E, Rassekh B, Gupta S, Perry H. A comprehensive review of the evidence regarding the effectiveness of Community-based Primary Health Care in improving maternal, neonatal, and child health: 4. child health findings. J Glob Health. 2017;7:010904.

33 Perry H, Rassekh B, Gupta S, Freeman P. A comprehensive review of the evidence regarding the effectiveness of community-based primary health care in improving maternal, neonatal and child health: 6. strategies used by effective projects. J Glob Health. 2017;7:010906.

34 Tanser F, Gijsbertsen B, Herbst K. Modelling and understanding primary health care accessibility and utilization in rural South Africa: an exploration using a Geographical Information System. Soc Sci Med. 2006;63:691-705. Medline:16574290 doi:10.1016/j.socscimed.2006.01.015

35 Houweling TA, Tripathy P, Nair N, Rath S, Rath S, Gope R, et al. The equity impact of participatory women's groups to reduce neonatal mortality in India: secondary analysis of a cluster-randomised trial. Int J Epidemiol. 2013;42:520-32. Medline:23509239 doi:10.1093/ije/dyt012

36 Valdivia M. Public health infrastructure and equity in the utilization of outpatient health care services in Peru. Health Policy Plan. 2002;17 Suppl:12-9. Medline:12477737 doi:10.1093/heapol/17.suppl_1.12

37 Alberts JF, Sanderman R, Eimers JM, van den Heuvel WJ. Heuler Wvd. Socioeconomic inequity in health care: a study of services utilization in Curaçao. Soc Sci Med. 1997;45:213-20. Medline:9225409 doi:10.1016/S0277-9536(96)00338-3

38 Bohren MA, Vogel J, Hunter E, Lutsiv O, Makh S, Souza JP, et al. The mistreatment of women during childbirth in health facilities globally: a mixed-methods systematic review. PLoS Med. 2015;12:e1001847. Medline:26126110 doi:10.1371/journal.pmed.1001847

39 Tappis H, Koblinsky M, Doocy S, Warren N, Peters D. Bypassing primary care facilities for childbirth: findngs from a multilevel analysis of skills birth attendance determinants in Afghanistan. J Midwifery Womens Health. 2016;61:185-95. Medline:26861932 doi:10.1111/jmwh.12359

40 Ahmed S, Khan MM. Is demand-side financing equity enhancing? Lessons from a maternal health voucher scheme in Bangladesh. Soc Sci Med. 2011;72:1704-10. Medline:21546145 doi:10.1016/j.socscimed.2011.03.031

41 Baqui AH, Rosecrans AM, Williams EK, Agarwal PK, Ahmed S, Darmstadt G. NGO facilitation of a government community-based maternal and neonatal health programme in rural India: improvements in equity. Health Policy Plan. 2008;23:234-43. Medline:18562458 doi:10.1093/heapol/czn012

42 Kumar V, Kumar A, Das V, Srivastava N, Baqui A, Darmstadt G. Community-driven impact of a newborn-focused behavioral intervention on maternal Health in Shivarg, India. Int J Gynaecol Obstet. 2012;117:48-55. Medline:22281244 doi:10.1016/j.ijgo.2011.10.031

43 World Bank. Analyzing Health Equity: Introduction. 2008. Available: https://openknowledge.worldbank.org/handle/10986/6896. Accessed: 26 April 2017.

44 Chopra M, Sharkey A, Dalmiya N, Anthony D, Birkin N. Strategies to improve health coverage and narrow the equity gap in child survival, health, and nutrition. Lancet. 2012;380:1331-40. Medline:22999430 doi:10.1016/S0140-6736(12)61423-8

45 Winestock Luna J, Monga T, Morgan L. Equity matters–lessons from MCHIP and CSHGP in Measuring and Improving Equity. Washington, DC: USAID/MCHIP, 2014.

46 Anderson LM, Adeney K, Shinn C, Safranek S, Buckner-Brown J, Krause LK. Community coalition-driven interventions to reduce health disparities among racial and ethnic minority populations. Cochrane Database Syst Rev. 2015;6:CD009905. Medline:26075988

47 Scheil-Adlung X. Global evidence on inequities in rural health protection: new data on rural deficits in health coverage for 174 countries. Extension of Social Security. 2015. Available: http://www.social-protection.org/gimi/gess/RessourcePDF.action?ressource.ressourceId=51297. Accessed: 26 April 2017.

48 Lassi Z, Kumar R, Bhutta Z. Community-based Care to Improve Maternal, Newborn, and Child Health. In: Black R, Laxminarayan R, Temmerman M, walker N, editors. Reproductive, Maternal, Newborn, and Child Health. 3rd ed. Washington DC; World Bank Group: 2016.

49 Ikeda N, Saito E, Kondo N, Inoue M, Ikeda S, Satoh T, et al. What has made the population of Japan Healthy? Lancet. 2011;378:1094-105. Medline:21885105 doi:10.1016/S0140-6736(11)61055-6

50 Rifkin SB. A framework linking community empowerment and health equity: it is a matter of CHOICE. J Health Popul Nutr. 2003;21:168-80. Medline:14717563

51 Victora CG, Wagstaff A, Schellenberg JA, Gwatkin D, Claeson M, Habicht J-P. Applying an equity lens to child health and mortality: more of the same is not enough. Lancet. 2003;362:233-41. Medline:12885488 doi:10.1016/S0140-6736(03)13917-7

52 Szwarcwald CL, Souza-Junior PR, Damacena GN. Socioeconomic inequalities in the use of outpatient services in Brazil according to health care need: evidence from the World Health Survey. BMC Health Serv Res. 2010;10:217. Medline:20653970 doi:10.1186/1472-6963-10-217

53 Malik SM, Ashraf N. Equity in the use of public services for mother and newborn child health care in Pakistan: a utilization incidence analysis. Int J Equity Health. 2016;15:120. Medline:27459961 doi:10.1186/s12939-016-0405-x

Acknowledgement: *originally published as: Meike Schleiff, Richard Kumapley, Paul A Freeman, Sundeep Gupta, Bahie M Rassekh, Henry B Perry:Comprehensive review of the evidence regarding the effectiveness of Community–Based Primary Health Care in improving maternal, neonatal and child health:5. equity effects for neonates and children. Reprinted with permission from Edinburgh University Global Health Society under Creative Commons Attribution Licence (Journal of Global Health 2017; 010905).*

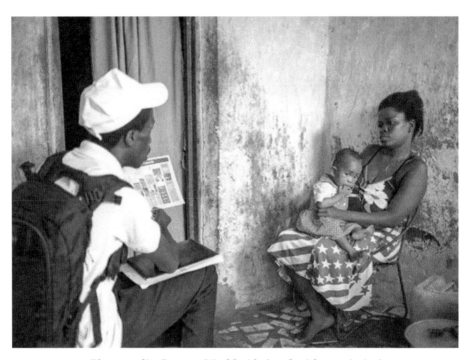

Photo credit: Concern Worldwide (used with permission).

Comprehensive review of the evidence regarding the effectiveness of community–based primary health care in improving maternal, neonatal and child health: 6. strategies used by effective projects

Henry B Perry[1], Emma Sacks[1], Meike Schleiff[1], Richard Kumapley[2], Sundeep Gupta[3], Bahie M Rassekh[4], Paul A Freeman[5,6]

[1] Department of International Health, Johns Hopkins Bloomberg School of Public Health, Baltimore, Maryland, USA
[2] UNICEF, New York, New York, USA
[3] Medical epidemiologist, Lusaka, Zambia
[4] The World Bank, Washington, District of Columbia, USA
[5] Independent consultant, Seattle, Washington, USA
[6] Department of Global Health, University of Washington, Seattle, Washington, USA

Background As part of our review of the evidence of the effectiveness of community–based primary health care (CBPHC) in improving maternal, neonatal and child health (MNCH), we summarize here the common delivery strategies of projects, programs and field research studies (collectively referred to as projects) that have demonstrated effectiveness in improving child mortality. Other articles in this series address specifically the effects of CBPHC on improving MNCH, while this paper explores the specific strategies used.

Methods We screened 12 166 published reports in PubMed of community–based approaches to improving maternal, neonatal and child health in high–mortality, resource–constrained settings from 1950–2015. A total of 700 assessments, including 148 reports from other publicly available sources (mostly unpublished evaluation reports and books) met the criteria for inclusion and were reviewed using a data extraction form. Here we identify and categorize key strategies used in project implementation.

Results Six categories of strategies for program implementation were identified, all of which required working in partnership with communities and health systems: (a) program design and evaluation, (b) community collaboration, (c) education for community–level staff, volunteers, beneficiaries and community members, (d) health systems strengthening, (e) use of community–level workers, and (f) intervention delivery. Four specific strategies for intervention delivery were identified: (a) recognition, referral, and (when possible) treatment of serious childhood illness by mothers and/or trained community agents, (b) routine systematic visitation of all homes, (c) facilitator–led participatory women's groups, and (d) health service provision at outreach sites by mobile health teams.

Conclusions The strategies identified here provide useful starting points for program design in strengthening the effectiveness of CBPHC for improving MNCH.

In recent decades, much of the funding for global health has concentrated on technical cooperation pertaining to strengthening narrowly focused vertical programs, such as control of HIV, malaria and tuberculosis, and expanding immunization coverage. However, in order to accelerate progress in the reduction of readily preventable deaths of children and mothers, there have been calls for more direct funding for integrated maternal and child health programs [1], health systems strengthening [2], integration of key interventions via a continuum of care [3,4], and stronger community participation [5]. However, none of these calls have sufficiently emphasized the importance of strengthening community–based service delivery strategies for accelerating progress by achieving high levels of coverage of evidence–based interventions. Too often, attention has been focused on the technical aspects of interventions rather than on the strategies and support systems that are needed to achieve high levels of population coverage.

Previous reviews have highlighted family and community practices that are important for maternal, newborn and child health [6] as well as specific technical interventions that can be provided in communities [7–10], but none have to date focused specifically on the implementation strategies that effective projects have used. This paper summarizes the various approaches used by the programs, projects and studies (hereafter referred to as projects) whose effectiveness has been assessed and included in a comprehensive database.

METHODS

We conducted a comprehensive review of the effectiveness of community–based primary health care (CBPHC) in improving maternal, newborn and child health (MNCH) by reviewing 12 186 published reports of community–based programs for improving MNCH in low– and middle–income countries. 552 of these reports qualified. An additional 148 reports were identified from the "grey" literature (documents publicly available on the internet) and books. A total of 700 assessments were included in this review. A full description of the search strategy and creation of the database is available elsewhere [11].

Of particular importance for this paper is that a data extraction form was designed to capture as much information as possible in the document containing the project's assessment that describes the project strategies and what role the community played. We did not attempt to force any strict definition of the term "community" in the analysis of the findings since there was no uniform definition used in the projects or by the reviewers. By strategies we mean the activities that these projects used to make the intervention effective – to plan the project, engage partners (including the community), implement the project, engage in associated activities not directly related to intervention delivery, and evaluate the project. The data extraction forms used to collect information from the assessments were designed to capture the available information regarding strategies used for project implementation. In particular, open–ended descriptions of project implementation were completed by reviewers.

A copy of the data extraction form is contained in Online Supplementary Document of the above–mentioned paper [11]. The form allows for open–ended as well as close–ended responses related to strategies and community engagement. Data were extracted from each assessment by two independent reviews and a third reviewer resolved any differences between the first two reviews.

The maternal, neonatal and child health database was searched carefully to identify all information that described the strategies that were used by projects. All available evidence in the database regarding strategies for project implementation was reviewed by reviewing all the open–responses individually and summarizing common themes as well as by adding up the number of responses to close–ended questions.

RESULTS

We identified six categories of strategies used by the projects in our database: (a) program design and evaluation, (b) community collaboration, (c) education for community–level staff, volunteers, beneficiaries and community members, (d) health systems strengthening, (e) use of community–level volunteers and workers (hereafter referred to as community health workers, or CHWs), and (f) intervention delivery. **Table 1** summarizes these strategies. The strategies were not mutually exclusive and most projects used at least several of these strategies and, in fact, some of the strategies fit into several categories (eg, participatory women's groups).

Strategies for program design and evaluation

Strategies for project design and evaluation shown in **Table 1** often included baseline and endline knowledge, practice and coverage (KPC) population–based household surveys. These made it possible to measure changes in inter-

Table 1. *Summary of strategies used by CBPHC projects to improve child health*

CATEGORY OF STRATEGY	SPECIFIC STRATEGY
Program design and evaluation	Knowledge, practice and coverage (KPC) household surveys
	Participatory Rural Appraisal (PRA)
	Village rosters of beneficiaries
	Census–taking
	Disease surveillance (based on information provided by community–based workers and communities)
	Prospective registration of vital events (pregnancies, births and deaths)
	Retrospective mortality assessment (based on maternal birth histories)
	Determination of cause of death from verbal autopsies
	Engagement of communities in planning and evaluation
Community engagement	Collaboration with or formation of village health committees and/or collaboration with local leaders
	Formation and/or support of women's groups
	Sharing locally obtained health–related data with the community
	Participatory Rural Appraisal (PRA)
	Formation and/or support of microcredit programs for women
	Involvement of older family members (men and grandparents/mothers–in–law)
Education of community–level staff, volunteers, beneficiaries and community members in general	Social marketing (media campaigns, posters, radio, etc.)
	Skits, stories and games for health education messages
	Peer–to–peer education (volunteer mothers visiting neighbors with targeted health messages)
	Education of grandmothers
	Positive deviance inquiry
	Training of trainers/cascade training
Health systems strengthening	Identification of cases of childhood illness in need of referral
	Strengthening referral system
	Strengthening of quality of care at referral facility
	Strengthening of supervisory system
	Strengthening logistics/drug supply system
	Training of providers at primary health center
	Training of community–level health care providers
Use of community health workers	Intermittent use of minimally trained volunteers for highly specific, targeted activities
	Use of volunteers for regular ongoing activities
	Use of trained and paid workers with 1–11 months of training
	Use of trained and paid workers with 1 year of training
Intervention delivery	Community case management
	Home visits
	Participatory women's groups
	Provision of health services at community outreach points by mobile teams from peripheral facilities

vention coverage in the program population as well as changes in childhood nutritional status as determined by anthropometry. Oftentimes, community members served as interviewers or collaborators for these surveys. In some projects, Participatory Rural Appraisal (PRA), an approach that incorporates the viewpoints of local people in the planning and management of development projects, was used to guide project planning or evaluation.

Various approaches were used to determine the beneficiary population (usually mothers, including pregnant women, and their young children) such as household censuses carried out by the project in collaboration with community members or the development of village rosters of beneficiaries. Sometimes projects included a disease–surveillance component using information provided by community–based workers and communities. Examples are surveillance for acute flaccid paralysis (to identify possible cases of polio) and for other vaccine–preventable diseases such as neonatal tetanus and measles. Some projects measured changes in mortality directly, either through prospective vital events registration as in Care Group projects [12] and in the pioneering CBPHC field project at Gadchiroli, India, conducted by SEARCH [13,14] or through retrospective measurements obtained from maternal birth histories [15,16]. Verbal autopsy methods have been used to assess the leading causes of child deaths in the project area and whether or not the cause of death "structure" has changed over time [17]. Finally, communities have been consulted during the project planning phase as well as at the time of project evaluation. In these circumstances, community members assist with data collection for structured surveys and participate as key informants or participants in focus group discussions.

Strategies for community engagement

Community engagement takes many forms and is commonly mentioned in the assessments included in our database (**Table 1**). Village health committees are often formed if they were not previously in existence, and projects work with them in project design, implementation and evaluation. Community leaders, including local religious leaders, are commonly consulted. Communities are often mobilized to participate in health campaigns or to practice key healthy behaviors. Many projects have worked with existing community groups or formed new ones, often women's groups. Activities that empower women are common forms of community engagement, including education and consciousness raising of women as well as formation and support of women's microcredit and savings groups.

Communities are commonly requested to participate in the selection of CHWs and to provide support to them and participate in their supervision. Finally, in some projects, special activities are geared toward engaging fathers, mothers–in–law, traditional healers and local drug sellers. Finally, though not commonly, projects have engaged communities by sharing surveillance and evaluation results. Noteworthy examples of projects with strong community engagement strategies include mobilization of churches in Mozambique [12] and Nigeria [18] and national mobilization of communities and short–term community workers for national health weeks in Sierra Leone [19].

Strategies for education of community–level staff, volunteers, beneficiaries and community members in general

Assessments of the effectiveness of projects included in our database have adopted many innovative approaches to educating CHWs, beneficiaries, and community members as a whole. Some have used social marketing channels such as radio and posters to convey key messages to the entire community. Others have conveyed health education messages through skits, puppet shows and games that engaged children, mothers, or the entire community. One noteworthy example of this approach is the World Relief child survival project in Cambodia [20,21].

Other approaches involved teaching health education messages to volunteer or paid community workers (who most often are mothers) who then conveyed them to their neighbors at the time of home visits or at meetings of small groups of neighbors. Sometimes projects targeted grandmothers for health education messages since they are respected and influential elders in the community. One particularly innovative educational strategy used in some projects is positive deviance inquiry, usually for addressing childhood undernutrition [22]. With this strategy, mothers of undernourished children in a village learn from the mothers of well–nourished children in the village how they care for their children – not just how they feed them but how they care for them more broadly.

Another approach used by some projects is called Care Groups [23], which involves training a small number of master trainers in a project area with a set of health education messages. These trainers each then train another set of trainers who then train another set. Through this "cascade training" approach, large numbers of peer–to–peer counselors can be trained to convey key messages to every household.

Strategies for health systems strengthening

Many CBPHC projects carried out health system strengthening activities of various sorts. One of the most common was providing mothers and their families with educational messages about warning signs for serious childhood illness or about pregnancy and childbirth for which care should be sought at a health facility. A stronger health system is one in which people seek care appropriately and, when potentially serious conditions are present, prompt care is sought. This is core feature of the approach known as Community–based Integrated Management of Childhood Illness (C–IMCI), utilized in many child survival projects funded by the US Agency for International Development, often with marked expansions of geographic coverage of key child survival interventions. A publication highlighting a number of these projects has been published [24].

Another approach has been to work with communities to establish emergency transport systems to ensure that mothers and children can access the nearest health facility whenever a complication arises and also ensure that the family can obtain transport at a fixed, fair, and affordable price. These referral systems are sometimes linked to insurance schemes whereby families pay small amounts of money on a regular basis, usually during pregnancy, to cover all or most of the cost of such transport if needed. One such approach has been developed by Curamericas for isolated mountainous communities in Guatemala [25,26].

Many projects, while implementing community–based interventions, also engage in activities to strengthen the quality of care provided at primary health care centers or referral hospitals, including the capacity of facilities to accept and care for referrals. This often takes the form of training staff who work there or helping the facility to improve its own stock of drugs and supplies.

Other approaches include improving the quality of the community–based health system itself by providing training to CHWs, by strengthening the supervision provided to CHWs, or strengthening the logistics/drug supply system for CHWs.

Strategies for use of community health workers

Community–based programs often rely on various types of CHWs – trained volunteers or more formally trained and paid workers who can implement specific interventions aimed at improving MNCH. The projects in our database engaged a broad variety of CHWs. For some projects, the training lasted only a few hours or days while for others CHWs had one year or more of full–time formal training. Some CHWs received only a "per diem" payment for attending a training course or a certificate for their service, while others were formally paid government employees. Some CHWs were volunteers or workers who had been engaged for a specific local project or study while others were part of a national government–run program.

Table 2 provides a listing and description of the types of CHWs described by reports in our database.

Strategies for implementation of interventions

Four types of strategies for implementing interventions were: (1) recognition, referral, and (in certain circumstances) treatment of serious childhood illness by mothers and/or CHWs; (2) routine systematic visitation of all homes, (3) facilitator–led participatory women's groups; and (4) provision of health services at community outreach points by mobile teams from peripheral facilities.

Community case management: recognition, referral, and (when possible) treatment of serious childhood illness by mothers and/or trained community agents

The review identified considerable evidence regarding the effectiveness of training and supervising CHWs to teach pregnant women and their families about danger signs during pregnancy and childbirth, during the newborn period, and among sick children [27–29]. CHWs can learn to recognize danger signs and they can teach these to mothers, other caregivers, and family members.

Table 2. *Specific examples of community health workers (CHWs) utilized in community–based primary health care (CBPHC) projects with evidence of effectiveness in improving neonatal and child health*

Category of CHW	Names given to CHWs in this category	Comment
Intermittent use of minimally trained unsalaried workers for highly specific, targeted activities	Child Health Day volunteer	May receive a per diem payment
Use of unsalaried workers for regular ongoing activities	Promoters, peer educators, malaria or nutrition agents, Care Group volunteers, animators, community case management workers, nutrition counselor mothers, bridge–to–health teams, family health workers, community surveillance volunteers, female community health volunteers	May receive certain incentives such as uniforms, per diem payment for training, or an occasional small stipend
Use of workers with 1–11 months of training who receive a salary	Health agents, community health agents, family planning agents, health surveillance assistants, *accompagnateurs*, lead mothers, *soccoristas*, Care Group facilitators (animators or promoters)	
Use of workers with 1 year or more of training who are salaried	Auxiliary nurses, community health officers, health extension workers	

Some projects that were effective in improving neonatal and child health also trained and supported CHWs to manage these conditions themselves (or in some cases these CHWs also taught mothers how to treat these conditions). This requires, in addition to proper training, appropriate supervision and logistical support for medications and other supplies [30–33]. The community–based treatment modalities included administration of oral (and in a few cases intramuscular) antibiotics [34], administration of oral rehydration fluids, provision of highly nutritious foods available locally or commercially prepared (known as ready–to–use therapeutic foods, or RUTF), and in some cases provision of micronutrients such as iron, vitamin A and zinc. When community–level workers did not have the capacity to treat children with acute illness, they informed mothers and caretakers that urgent treatment at a referral health facility was needed. A comprehensive manual for community–based diagnosis and treatment of serious childhood illness is available for general use [35]. Integrated community case management (iCCM) for childhood illness is now being scaled up in many countries [36].

Routine systematic visitation of homes

Routine systematic visitation of homes makes it possible to identify those in need of basic services and to provide everyone in the program population with essential health education and selected key services, particularly during pregnancy and the early neonatal period. Community–level workers who make home visits are generally able to identify pregnant women and mothers of young children, provide education to them and other family members (especially husbands and mothers–in–law), recognize danger signs during pregnancy and childhood illness, encourage referral when danger signs are present, and provide treatment for certain conditions that can be identified at the time of home visits such as growth faltering, diarrhea, pneumonia, and malaria.

Based on current evidence, the World Health Organization and UNICEF recommend that all pregnant women receive two home visits during the prenatal period, one home visit during the first 24 hours after birth, and at least one visit as soon as possible after delivery [37]. Activities that should take place during these visits include the following: education about proper nutrition, promotion of antenatal care, education about danger signs during pregnancy and childbirth, promotion of breastfeeding immediately after birth, prevention of hypothermia, and measurement of the weight of newborns to identify low–birth–weight newborns who need additional home visits. A number of studies have highlighted the difficulties many women face in accessing health facilities due to distance and cost [38]. Home visitation provides an alternative for those without ready access to health facilities.

Home visitation is also an effective means of providing counseling about breastfeeding and appropriate complementary feeding, hand washing, prevention and treatment of diarrhea, detection and treatment of childhood pneumonia, and family planning services. There are a number of variations of home visitation strategies using community–level workers, from weekly home visits for providing micronutrients to children [39] to regular monthly visitation of all homes in a program population as part of a more comprehensive approach to delivering basic services to the entire population [40].

Finally, an ongoing program of home visitation provides a foundation of trust and awareness. When children develop signs of serious illness that can be managed by CHWs (such as for pneumonia, diarrhea or malaria), families will be more predisposed to contact the CHW for early and prompt treatment.

Participatory women's groups

Participatory women's groups are led by facilitators with less than two weeks of training who provide the opportunity for further empowerment and education about healthy behaviors, danger signs of serious illness, and proper care of the newborn. These groups may also address issues outside of the health domain that are a priority to the community and that may also have an indirect effect on health (such as income generation activities). These groups may also provide a vehicle for counseling about breastfeeding, birth spacing, infant feeding, hand washing, prevention and treatment of diarrhea, signs of childhood pneumonia, and danger signs during pregnancy and childbirth. Participatory women's groups also can be effective for assisting mothers to rehabilitate malnourished children detected through growth monitoring.

The literature illustrates several effective approaches to facilitating participatory women's groups, including the use of a participatory action–learning cycle [41,42], formation of Care Groups (10–15 women volunteers who meet with a facilitator (promoter/animator) once a month to learn a key health education message to disseminate to each of the mothers in the 10–15 households surrounding each volunteer) [43,44], and education sessions led by community mobilizers [45].

Provision of services at satellite clinics, including holding outreach immunization sessions, by mobile teams from peripheral facilities

Provision of services at satellite clinics, including holding outreach immunization sessions, by mobile teams based at health centers is a common means of community–based outreach. These mobile teams may have a vehicle or more likely a motorcycle, bicycle, horse or donkey, or they may even travel by foot. The provision of immunization services by mobile health teams at points beyond a peripheral health facility is now well–developed in many low–income countries [46]. Other examples of services that can be provided through outreach include promotion of and provision of family planning services, basic antenatal care, testing for HIV and syphilis, distribution of insecticide–treated bed nets, distribution of medications to prevent or treat malaria, and growth monitoring to detect cases of childhood malnutrition.

One widely implemented variation of this strategy is Child Health Days (or sometimes called Child Health Weeks). Generally occurring twice a year, they usually include some combination of immunization administration, vitamin A supplementation, nutritional monitoring (and referral of malnourished children), and distribution of oral rehydration packets, water–purification tablets, or de–worming tablets [47,48]. Services are provided at peripheral outreach points separate from a health center such as at a school or community building or even under a tree, and home visits are often carried out in addition to reach those mothers and children who did not come to the outreach points. These children are often identified on the basis of previously developed household registers.

Table 3 demonstrates which evidence–based child survival interventions can be implemented by which implementation modality. The interventions shown in **Table 3** are those which have been identified by the Lives Saved Tool (LiST) for inclusion in program plans for reducing under–5 mortality [49]. A more detailed discussion of these four intervention delivery strategies has been reported elsewhere [50].

Frequency of selected program–related processes

When program assessments that qualified for the review underwent data extraction, reviewers were asked to describe the degree to which communities were involved in various aspects of the project. Some of the findings are contained in **Table 4**. These findings demonstrate a high degree of community engagement, both in the maternal as well as the neonatal/child health CBPHC projects. More than three–fourths of the projects trained CHWs and more than one–third engaged communities in the formation or support of community groups as well as in the planning of project activities. 81% of the projects engaged communities in project implementation, and more than half promoted partnerships between the community and the health program, promoted the use of local resources, or promoted community empowerment. Almost half promoted women's empowerment, one–third promoted leadership in the community, and one–quarter promoted equity. 40% of the projects involved

Table 3. *Child health interventions with strong evidence of effectiveness through community–based implementation*

TECHNICAL INTERVENTION	COMMUNITY–BASED INTERVENTION DELIVERY STRATEGY			
	Community case management	Home visits	Participatory women's groups	Outreach services
Immunizations: BCG, polio, diphtheria, pertussis, tetanus, measles, Haemophilus Influenza Type b (Hib), pneumococcus, rotavirus immunizations for children; tetanus immunization for mothers and women of reproductive age		X		X
Provision of supplemental vitamin A to children 6–59 months of age and to post–partum mothers		X		X
Provision of preventive zinc supplements to all children 6–59 months of age		X		X
Promotion of breastfeeding immediately after birth, exclusive breastfeeding during the first 6 months of life and continued non–exclusive breastfeeding beyond 6 months	X	X	X	X
Promotion of appropriate complementary feeding beginning at 6 months of age	X	X	X	X
Promotion of hygiene (including hand washing), safe water, and sanitation	X	X	X	X
Promotion of oral rehydration therapy (ORT) for diarrhea with or without zinc supplementation	X	X	X	X
Promotion of clean deliveries, especially where most births occur at home and hygiene is poor		X	X	X
Detection/referral of pneumonia with or without provision of community–based treatment	X	X	X	X
Home–based neonatal care (frequent home visits for promotion of immediate and exclusive breastfeeding, promotion of cleanliness, prevention of hypothermia, and diagnosis and treatment of neonatal sepsis by CHW)	X	X	X	
Community–based rehabilitation of children with protein–calorie undernutrition through food supplementation (including rehabilitation of children with severe acute undernutrition through ready–to–use dry therapeutic foods)	X	X	X	X
Insecticide–treated bed nets (ITNs) in malaria–endemic areas		X	X	X
Indoor residual spraying in malaria–endemic areas		X		X
Detection/referral of malaria with or without provision of community–based treatment	X	X	X	X
Intermittent preventive treatment of malaria during pregnancy (IPTp) and infancy (IPTi) in malaria–endemic areas		X		X
Detection and treatment of syphilis in pregnant women in areas of high prevalence		X		X
Promotion of HIV testing in pregnant women and prevention of mother–to–child transmission (PMTCT) of HIV infection	X	X	X	X
Iodine supplementation in iodine–deficient areas where fortified salt is not consumed		X	X	X
Provision and promotion of family planning services		X	X	X

*Outreach of health facility staff includes holding mobile clinics and/or immunization sessions at specified locations outside of health facilities in outlying communities on a regular basis.

Table 4. *Community involvement in the implementation of maternal, neonatal and child health CBPHC projects included in the database*

STAGE OF IMPLE-MENTA-TION	ACTIVITY	PERCENTAGE OF ASSESSMENTS OF MATERNAL CBPHC PROJ-ECTS THAT DE-SCRIBE ACTIVITY (N = 152)	PERCENTAGE OF ASSESSMENTS OF NEONATAL AND/OR CHILD HEALTH CBPHC PROJECTS THAT DESCRIBE ACTIVITY (N = 548)	PERCENTAGE OF ASSESS-MENTS OF ALL MATER-NAL, NEONATAL AND/OR CHILD HEALTH CBPHC PROJECTS COMBINED THAT DESCRIBE ACTIV-ITY (N = 700)
Inputs	Training of CHWs	86.3	74.0	76.6
	Formation and/or support of community groups	53.6	35.5	39.5
	Community involvement in planning	46.4	36.1	38.3
Processes	Community involvement in implementation	90.8	78.1	80.9
	Promotion of partnerships between the community and the health program	73.2	53.6	57.8
	Promotion of the use of local resources	74.5	53.2	57.8
	Promotion of community empowerment	62.7	53.6	55.6
	Promotion of leadership in the community	41.8	30.4	32.9
	Promotion of women's empowerment	62.7	40.6	45.4
	Promotion of equity	24.8	24.8	24.8
Evaluation	Community involvement in evaluation	50.3	37.5	40.3

the community in the project evaluation. These findings are highly likely to underestimate the true situation since a large portion of the assessments did not go into this level of detail in describing the community engagement component of the project. Information provided in the assessment was rarely sufficient to provide any deeper understanding of the quality of community engagement or details of how community engagement was actually carried out.

DISCUSSION

This analysis of strategies used by effective community–based programs for improving MNCH has documented a high degree of community engagement in project implementation. Six categories of strategies were identified: (a) program design and evaluation, (b) community collaboration, (c) education for community–level staff, volunteers, beneficiaries and community members, (d) health systems strengthening, (e) use of CHWs, and (f) intervention delivery. Within each strategy category, community engagement was an essential element for strategy implementation. By its very nature, CPBHC requires community engagement for virtually all aspects of programming. Each of these aspects of community engagement are part of the process of building capacity within the community for the benefit of the health program and its capacity to improve the health of mothers, neonates and children. Further elaboration of these strategies as they pertain specifically to maternal, neonatal and child health are discussed in other articles in this series [51–53].

In general, the details of community–based strategies and approaches used by projects to improve MNCH have not been well described in the peer–reviewed scientific literature, where the focus is usually on the health impact of the intervention, or set of interventions, rather than on describing in sufficient detail the exact implementation strategies used to achieve that impact. The findings of this review provide insights into the richness of this dimension of implementation strategies and its importance for program effectiveness. **Figure 1** contains a framework that attempts to capture the importance of community empowerment for improving the health of mothers, neonates and children. The delivery process, along with the technical content of the interventions, is embedded in the eventual health outcomes produced together by the health system working with the community.

The framework in **Figure 1** and in fact the strategies identified in this article as well as the interventions identified in other articles in this series all highlight the importance of community engagement and community–based delivery of interventions outside of health facilities in order to reach those who need services. As Gwatkin et al. observed in their 1980 comprehensive review of the effectiveness of programs improving child health and nutrition [54]:

"Unless services reach those in need, even the best–conceived primary health and nutrition care programs can obviously have little impact on mortality. Thus, … the development of plans for getting services to the people is as important as are decisions concerning which services should be offered."

CBPHC involves, above all, getting services to those who need them.

Figure 1 emphasizes the importance of context. In fact, strategies in general are context– specific. In order for community–based programs to be successful, the context must be carefully considered in order to select the most appropriate combinations of interventions and implementation strategies. Program effec-

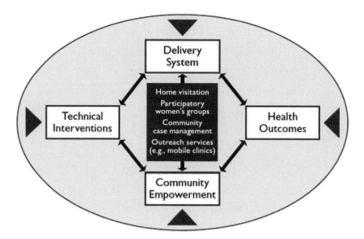

Figure 1. *A conceptual framework for planning, implementing and evaluating community–based primary health care programs for improving maternal, neonatal and child health. Blue triangles represent contextual factors.*

tiveness in improving MNCH in a given geographical area requires knowing the local epidemiological priorities (ie, the most frequent and readily preventable or treatable serious conditions) as well as the feasibility of achieving high coverage of evidence–based interventions targeting the epidemiological priorities given the available resources, logistical challenges, contextual constraints (including health system constraints), and available implementation strategies.

The assessments making up our database are derived largely from small demonstration projects, short–term trials, and efficacy studies of one or a small number of interventions. More independent, rigorous assessments of large–scale integrated programs at scale carried out for five or more years are needed. There are few examples of rigorous assessments of CBPHC at scale over a longer time period. However, these few studies show that the bottlenecks to the effectiveness of large–scale programs include assuring that the number of CHWs and their supervisors is sufficient for the population being served, and that CHWs receive adequate support and supervision, including the basic commodities they need to do their work [55,56]. Future research is needed to rigorously assess the effectiveness of community–based approaches at scale in relatively routine conditions [57].

Elsewhere in this series we review the common characteristics of four projects that have long–term evidence of effectiveness [58]. A more in–depth analysis of the strategies and effectiveness of the larger projects included in our review has not been carried out. Although such an analysis would be useful, unfortunately it is beyond the scope of the current series of articles. Questions that might be addressed through such an analysis include:

- Is effectiveness weakened as projects scale up? If not, what specific steps were taken to maintain quality and effectiveness?
- What kinds of community engagement and what kinds of community–level workers were used in different projects, and how did these features contribute to effectiveness?
- What is the contribution of civil society and NGOs to larger–scale projects and how do these contributions affect the effectiveness of public–sector programs?

Health programs need to ensure that local health facilities are appropriately staffed and that the staff has the training, equipment, supplies and transport needed to support community–level work. For example, mobile health teams based at peripheral facilities need, at a minimum, steady supplies of vaccines and adequate transport. Additionally, compassionate and high–quality curative and referral care, including basic hospital and surgical care, lends credibility to the community–based work and the workers who provide it. Small, well–run first–level referral hospitals can be cost–effective in improving health and can serve as an important asset for the community to gain trust in the health system [59,60].

Health systems can benefit greatly from having a community–level worker implement evidence–based interventions in order to achieve high population coverage of these interventions. One recent analysis [61] concluded that almost two–thirds (59%) of maternal, prenatal, neonatal, and child deaths that could be prevented by all currently available interventions could be prevented with community–based approaches. Facility–based approaches would avert far fewer (20% at primary health care centers and 22% at hospitals).

Of course, the community–level workers who implement these interventions in collaboration with communities must be appropriately trained and supported; a recent Cochrane Review identified the need for adequate and standardized compensation or incentives for CHWs [62]. An effective strategy must be developed for promptly selecting and training new CHWs to replace those who are no longer functioning in this capacity. Although these decisions are normally made by program leaders in consultation with local communities, examples exist in which communities have taken full responsibility for this process [63]. In addition to continuing research on the capability of CHWs to provide specific interventions, more research will be needed on how many interventions a given CHW can take on and what training and supervision are required to maintain quality.

As we have seen in this analysis, empowering the community to be a partner with the health system can help strengthen community–based delivery strategies, as described in **Figure 1**. The finding supports the recent assertion of Marston et al. [64] that community participation (in which communities work together with health services for the co–production of health care) will be central for achieving the recently released World Health Organization global strategy for women's and children's health [65].

Community case management, routine systematic home visitation, participatory women's groups, and outreach services provided by mobile teams represent important delivery strategies for improving MNCH in high–mortality, resource–constrained settings. These strategies are not the only approaches to implementing interventions that can improve child health, but they are the most common strategies used in the projects whose assessments are included in our database.

Routine systematic home visitation has the unique advantage of not only delivering key interventions to all who need them but also of ensuring that no one is left out. Marginalization and discrimination of sub–groups in high–mortality, resource–constrained settings are not uncommon, leading to many social barriers – in addition to geographic barriers – in accessing services at facilities or even at peripheral outreach points. Thus, for instance, home visits have proven to be an essential strategy for the final stages of polio eradication [66].

Cesar Victora, one of the widely acknowledged leaders of the global movement to improve MNCH, lamented that "We have the bullets [interventions] but not the guns [implementation strategies]" for a second child survival revolution [67]. The analysis provided here helps to point the way forward by identifying implementation strategies used by programs with demonstrated effectiveness.

Study limitations

The word limits placed on peer–reviewed journal articles make it difficult to fully describe implementation strategies. Our data extraction process was set up to glean whatever information was available regarding these strategies. Our database has been strengthened by the inclusion of 116 assessments that are not peer–reviewed journal articles, and many of them describe their strategies in greater detail. Most of these additional 116 assessments are either unpublished evaluation reports that are publicly available or books. These documents are useful in part because they are not subject to the same space limitations as peer–reviewed articles and can provide more information. Further consolidation and analysis of the extensive and rich evidence about strategies for implementation of CBPHC projects described in the gray literature (including a rigorous examination of the quality of the assessments) would be useful but goes beyond the capacity of the current series of articles to address.

Another limitation of this study is that some of the findings reported here are based on subjective judgments of reviewers. However, the procedure we used – having each assessment reviewed independently by two researchers and then having a third resolve any differences – helps to mitigate this limitation.

A final limitation of our review is the overall difficulty of assessing community participation and engagement. While one of the strengths of our paper is highlighting and further describing the role of the community in implementing effective CBPHC projects, we also note that frameworks and indicators for assessing the quality and effectiveness of this critical dimension of CBPHC were rarely used in the assessments included in our review. Appropriate frameworks and indicators need to be used by future CBPHC projects so that they can more fully describe the role of the community in the process of implementation and better assess the contribution that this made to health outcomes. Useful and more robust approaches to describing and analyzing the process of community participation are available [68,69].

CONCLUSIONS

This analysis provides an overview of the ways in which CBPHC projects have planned and evaluated their activities, how they collaborated with communities, how they have used CHWs, and how they have strengthened health systems. The evidence from this review supports the proposition that the application of these strategies can accelerate the decline in maternal, neonatal and child mortality in priority countries. These strategies require that the health system establish functional partnerships with community leaders and community members in order to achieve high levels of coverage of evidence–based interventions. Building the capacity of health systems to work with communities to implement these strategies is one of the priority tasks for ending preventable child and maternal deaths by 2030.

Using the strategies identified here for strengthening CBPHC to improve MNCH can establish an entry point for developing synergies with community–based approaches for the detection and treatment of HIV/AIDS [70], tuberculosis [71] and malaria [31] as well as for the promotion of family planning services [72], detection and treatment of adult non–communicable diseases [73], and the achievement of universal health coverage. This review supports the growing recognition that community–based programs in high–mortality, resource–constrained settings have a great potential for improving MNCH at low cost.

Nonetheless, awareness about the full potential of CBPHC is still not yet widespread, and evidence of the effectiveness of CBPHC at scale in priority settings remains limited. Determining the fit and feasibility, within existing local and health systems constraints, of CBPHC implementation strategies for MNCH interventions is a pressing challenge for national programs. Unleashing the full potential of communities as partners in the process of building effective health systems in high–mortality, resource–constrained settings is one of the great frontiers for global health in the 21st century.

Acknowledgments: We are grateful to Melanie Morrow for her review of an earlier draft of this paper. We are grateful to the following organizations that provided small grants to cover the expenses of this review: UNICEF, the World Bank, the Department of Child and Adolescent Health and Development of the World Health Organization, the CORE Group (Collaboration and Resources for Child Health)/USAID, Future Generations, and the Gates Foundation. We are also grateful to the American Public Health Association and particularly its International Health Section staff, which administered some of these funds. We thank Future Generations for providing office space, administrative support, and salary support to Dr Perry during the initial phase of the review. The World Bank made it possible for one of its consultants, Dr Bahie Rassekh, to participate as a member of the Study Team.

Funding: *The following organizations provided funds that were used to conduct the work described in this article: The World Health Organization, UNICEF, the World Bank, the United States Agency for International Development, and the Gates Foundation. The organizations that provided financial support had no role in the execution of the review.*

Authorship declaration: *HP wrote the first draft. HP, PF, BR, and SG guided this project from the beginning to the end and participated in all decisions related to the overall review. ES and RK performed the analysis of the quantitative data included in our report. All of the authors participated in the revision of earlier drafts and approved the final draft.*

Competing interests: *All authors have completed the Unified Competing Interest Form at www.icmje.org/coi_disclosure.pdf (available upon request from the corresponding author), and declare no conflict of interest.*

References

1 World Health Organization, Organisation for Economic Co-operation and Development, World Bank. Effective Aid, Better Health. Geneva: World Health Organization, 2008.

2 Reich MR, Takemi K. G8 and strengthening of health systems: follow-up to the Toyako summit. Lancet. 2009;373:508-15. Medline:19150128 doi:10.1016/S0140-6736(08)61899-1

3 Bhutta ZA, Ali S, Cousens S, Ali TM, Haider BA, Rizvi A, et al. Alma-Ata: Rebirth and revision 6–interventions to address maternal, newborn, and child survival: what difference can integrated primary health care strategies make? Lancet. 2008;372:972-89. Medline:18790320 doi:10.1016/S0140-6736(08)61407-5

4 Ekman B, Pathmanathan I, Liljestrand J. Integrating health interventions for women, newborn babies, and children: a framework for action. Lancet. 2008;372:990-1000. Medline:18790321 doi:10.1016/S0140-6736(08)61408-7

5 Rosato M, Laverack G, Grabman LH, Tripathy P, Nair N, Mwansambo C, et al. Community participation: lessons for maternal, newborn, and child health. Lancet. 2008;372:962-71. Medline:18790319 doi:10.1016/S0140-6736(08)61406-3

6 Hill Z, Kirkwood B, Edmond KM. Family and community practices that promote child survival, growth and development: a review of the evidence. Geneva, Switzerland: World Health Organization; 2004.

7 Bhutta ZA, Darmstadt GL, Hasan BS, Haws RA. Community-based interventions for improving perinatal and neonatal health outcomes in developing countries: a review of the evidence. Pediatrics. 2005;115:519-617. Medline:15866863 doi:10.1542/peds.2004-1441

8 Darmstadt GL, Bhutta ZA, Cousens S, Adam T, Walker N, de Bernis L. Evidence-based, cost-effective interventions: how many newborn babies can we save? Lancet. 2005;365:977-88. Medline:15767001 doi:10.1016/S0140-6736(05)71088-6

9 Bhutta ZA, Ahmed T, Black RE, Cousens S, Dewey K, Giugliani E, et al. What works? Interventions for maternal and child undernutrition and survival. Lancet. 2008;371:417-40. Medline:18206226 doi:10.1016/S0140-6736(07)61693-6

10 Jones G, Steketee RW, Black RE, Bhutta ZA, Morris SS. How many child deaths can we prevent this year? Lancet. 2003;362:65-71. Medline:12853204 doi:10.1016/S0140-6736(03)13811-1

11 Perry H, Rassekh B, Gupta S, Wilhelm J, Freeman P. A comprehensive review of the evidence regarding the effectiveness of community-based primary health care in improving maternal, neonatal and child health: 1. rationale, methods and database description. J Glob Health. 2017;7:010901.

12 Edward A, Ernst P, Taylor C, Becker S, Mazive E, Perry H. Examining the evidence of under-five mortality reduction in a community-based programme in Gaza, Mozambique. Trans R Soc Trop Med Hyg. 2007;101:814-22. Medline:17482222 doi:10.1016/j.trstmh.2007.02.025

13 Bang AT, Bang RA, Tale O, Sontakke P, Solanki J, Wargantiwar R, et al. Reduction in pneumonia mortality and total childhood mortality by means of community-based intervention trial in Gadchiroli, India. Lancet. 1990;336:201-6. Medline:1973770 doi:10.1016/0140-6736(90)91733-Q

14 Bang AT, Bang RA, Reddy HM. Home-based neonatal care: summary and applications of the field trial in rural Gadchiroli, India (1993 to 2003). J Perinatol. 2005;25 Suppl 1:S108-22. Medline:15791272 doi:10.1038/sj.jp.7211278

15 Perry H, Berggren W, Berggren G, Dowell D, Menager H, Bottex E, et al. Long-term reductions in mortality among children under age 5 in rural Haiti: effects of a comprehensive health system in an impoverished setting. Am J Public Health. 2007;97:240-6. Medline:17194853 doi:10.2105/AJPH.2006.088732

16 Johnson AD, Thomson DR, Atwood S, Alley I, Beckerman JL, Kone I, et al. Assessing early access to care and child survival during a health system strengthening intervention in Mali: a repeated cross sectional survey. PLoS One. 2013;8:e81304. Medline:24349053 doi:10.1371/journal.pone.0081304

17 Perry HB, Shanklin DS, Schroeder DG. Impact of a community-based comprehensive primary healthcare programme on infant and child mortality in Bolivia. J Health Popul Nutr. 2003;21:383-95. Medline:15038594

18 Ezeanolue EE, Obiefune MC, Ezeanolue CO, Ehiri JE, Osuji A, Ogidi AG, et al. Effect of a congregation-based intervention on uptake of HIV testing and linkage to care in pregnant women in Nigeria (Baby Shower): a cluster randomised trial. Lancet Glob Health. 2015;3:e692-700. Medline:26475016 doi:10.1016/S2214-109X(15)00195-3

19 Sesay FF, Hodges MH, Kamara HI, Turay M, Wolfe A, Samba TT, et al. High coverage of vitamin A supplementation and measles vaccination during an integrated Maternal and Child Health Week in Sierra Leone. Int Health. 2015;7:26-31. Medline:25316706 doi:10.1093/inthealth/ihu073

20 Relief W. "Light for Life" Child Survival Project, Kampong Cam Province (Cambodia): Final Evaluation (2003-2007). Baltimore, MD: World Relief, 2007.

21 Perry H, Sivan O, Bowman G, Casazza L, Edward A, Hansen K, et al. Averting childhood deaths in resource-constrained settings through engagement with the community: an example from Cambodia. In: Gofin J, Gofin R, editors. Essentials of Community Health. Sudbury, MA: Jones and Bartlett; 2010.

22 Berggren G. Nutritional Education and rehabilitation Program: A Save the Children Project in Vietnam. In: Wollinka O, Keeley E, Burkhalter RB, Bashir N, editors. The Hearth Nutrition Model: Applications in Haiti, Vietnam, and Bangladesh. Wheaton, Il, and Arlington, VA: World Relief and BASICS; 1997.

23 Perry H, Morrow M, Borger S, Weiss J, DeCoster M, Davis T, et al. Care Groups I: An innovative community-based strategy for improving maternal, neonatal, and child health in resource-constrained settings. Glob Health Sci Pract. 2015;3:358-69. Medline:26374798 doi:10.9745/GHSP-D-15-00051

24 Ricca J, Kureshy N, Leban K, Prosnitz D, Ryan L. Community-based intervention packages facilitated by NGOs demonstrate plausible evidence for child mortality impact. Health Policy Plan. 2014;29:204-16. Medline:23434515 doi:10.1093/heapol/czt005

25 Global C. Focused Strategic Assessment: USAID Child Survival and Health Grants Program "Community-Based, Impact-Oriented Child Survival in Huehuetenango, Guatemala". 2015. Available: http://www.mcsprogram.org/wp-content/uploads/2016/09/Curamericas_Guatemala_FE.pdf. Accessed: 26 April 2017.

26 Stollak I, Valdez M, Rivas K, Perry H. Casas Maternas in the Rural Highlands of Guatemala: a mixed-methods case study of the introduction and utilization of birthing facilities by an indigenous population. Glob Health Sci Pract. 2016;4:114-31. Medline:27016548 doi:10.9745/GHSP-D-15-00266

27 Bang AT, Reddy HM, Deshmukh MD, Baitule SB, Bang RA. Neonatal and infant mortality in the ten years (1993 to 2003) of the Gadchiroli field trial: effect of home-based neonatal care. J Perinatol. 2005;25 Suppl 1:S92-107. Medline:15791283 doi:10.1038/sj.jp.7211277

28 Baqui AH, El-Arifeen S, Darmstadt GL, Ahmed S, Williams EK, Seraji HR, et al. Effect of community-based newborn-care intervention package implemented through two service-delivery strategies in Sylhet district, Bangladesh: a cluster-randomised controlled trial. Lancet. 2008;371:1936-44. Medline:18539225 doi:10.1016/S0140-6736(08)60835-1

29 Kumar V, Mohanty S, Kumar A, Misra RP, Santosham M, Awasthi S, et al. Effect of community-based behaviour change management on neonatal mortality in Shivgarh, Uttar Pradesh, India: a cluster-randomised controlled trial. Lancet. 2008;372:1151-62. Medline:18926277 doi:10.1016/S0140-6736(08)61483-X

30 Baqui AH, Arifeen SE, Williams EK, Ahmed S, Mannan I, Rahman SM, et al. Effectiveness of home-based management of newborn infections by community health workers in rural Bangladesh. Pediatr Infect Dis J. 2009;28:304-10. Medline:19289979 doi:10.1097/INF.0b013e31819069e8

31 Kidane G, Morrow RH. Teaching mothers to provide home treatment of malaria in Tigray, Ethiopia: a randomised trial. Lancet. 2000;356:550-5. Medline:10950232 doi:10.1016/S0140-6736(00)02580-0

32 Sazawal S, Black RE. Effect of pneumonia case management on mortality in neonates, infants, and preschool children: a meta-analysis of community-based trials. Lancet Infect Dis. 2003;3:547-56. Medline:12954560 doi:10.1016/S1473-3099(03)00737-0

33 Chowdhury AMR, Cash RA. A Simple Solution: Teaching Millions to Treat Diarrhoea at Home. Dhaka, Bangladesh: University Press Limited; 1996.

34 Coffey PS, Sharma J, Gargi KC, Neupane D, Dawson P, Pradhan YV. Feasibility and acceptability of gentamicin in the Uniject prefilled injection system for community-based treatment of possible neonatal sepsis: the experience of female community health volunteers in Nepal. J Perinatol. 2012;32:959-65. Medline:22422117 doi:10.1038/jp.2012.20

35 CORE Group. Save the Children, BASICS. Community case management essentials: Treating common childhood illnesses in the community. A guide for program managers. Washington, DC: CORE Group; 2010. Available: http://www.coregroup.org/storage/documents/CCM/CCMbook-internet2.pdf. Accessed: 3 April 2017.

36 Young M, Wolfheim C, Marsh DR, Hammamy D. World Health Organization/United Nations Children's Fund Joint Statement on Integrated Community Case Management: an equity-focused strategy to improve access to essential treatment services for children. Am J Trop Med Hyg. 2012;87:6-10. Medline:23136272 doi:10.4269/ajtmh.2012.12-0221

37 WHO. UNICEF. WHO/UNICEF Joint Statement: Home Visits for the Newborn Child: A Strategy to Improve Survival. 2009. Available: http://apps.who.int/iris/bitstream/10665/70002/1/WHO_FCH_CAH_09.02_eng.pdf. Accessed: 26 April 2017.

38 Tanser F, Gijsbertsen B, Herbst K. Modelling and understanding primary health care accessibility and utilization in rural South Africa: an exploration using a geographical information system. Soc Sci Med. 2006;63:691-705. Medline:16574290 doi:10.1016/j.socscimed.2006.01.015

39 Baqui AH, Zaman K, Persson LA, El Arifeen S, Yunus M, Begum N, et al. Simultaneous weekly supplementation of iron and zinc is associated with lower morbidity due to diarrhea and acute lower respiratory infection in Bangladeshi infants. J Nutr. 2003;133:4150-7. Medline:14652364

40 Perry H, Cayemittes M, Philippe F, Dowell D, Dortonne JR, Menager H, et al. Reducing under-five mortality through Hopital Albert Schweitzer's integrated system in Haiti. Health Policy Plan. 2006;21:217-30. Medline:16565151 doi:10.1093/heapol/czl005

41 Prost A, Colbourn T, Seward N, Azad K, Coomarasamy A, Copas A, et al. Women's groups practising participatory learning and action to improve maternal and newborn health in low-resource settings: a systematic review and meta-analysis. Lancet. 2013;381:1736-46. Medline:23683640 doi:10.1016/S0140-6736(13)60685-6

42 Manandhar DS, Osrin D, Shrestha BP, Mesko N, Morrison J, Tumbahangphe KM, et al. Effect of a participatory intervention with women's groups on birth outcomes in Nepal: cluster-randomised controlled trial. Lancet. 2004;364:970-9. Medline:15364188 doi:10.1016/S0140-6736(04)17021-9

43 Perry H, Morrow M, Borger S, Weiss J, DeCoster M, Davis T, et al. Care Groups I: an emerging innovative community-based delivery strategy for improving maternal, neonatal and child health in high-mortality, resource-constrained settings. Glob Health Sci Pract. 2015;3:358-69. Medline:26374798 doi:10.9745/GHSP-D-15-00051

44 Perry H, Morrow M, Davis T, Borger S, Weiss J, DeCoster M, et al. Care Groups II: a summary of the maternal, neonatal and child health outcomes achieved in high-mortality, resource-constrained settings. Glob Health Sci Pract. 2015;3:370-81. Medline:26374799 doi:10.9745/GHSP-D-15-00052

45 Bhutta ZA, Memon ZA, Soofi S, Salat MS, Cousens S, Martines J. Implementing community-based perinatal care: results from a pilot study in rural Pakistan. Bull World Health Organ. 2008;86:452-9. Medline:18568274 doi:10.2471/BLT.07.045849

46 UNICEF. Tracking Progress in Maternal, Newborn and Child Survival. 2008. Available: http://www.who.int/pmnch/Countdownto2015FINALREPORT-apr7.pdf/. Accessed:26 April 2017.

47 Doherty T, Chopra M, Tomlinson M, Oliphant N, Nsibande D, Mason J. Moving from vertical to integrated child health programmes: experiences from a multi-country assessment of the Child Health Days approach in Africa. Trop Med Int Health. 2010;15:296-305. Medline:20070638 doi:10.1111/j.1365-3156.2009.02454.x

48 Palmer AC, Diaz T, Noordam AC, Dalmiya N. Evolution of the child health day strategy for the integrated delivery of child health and nutrition services. Food Nutr Bull. 2013;34:412-9. Medline:24605691 doi:10.1177/156482651303400406

49 Walker N, Tam Y, Friberg IK. Overview of the Lives Saved Tool (LiST). BMC Public Health. 2013;13 Suppl 3:S1. Medline:24564438 doi:10.1186/1471-2458-13-S3-S1

50 Perry H, Freeman P, Gupta S, Rassekh B. Building on the current evidence to strengthen community-based service delivery strategies for promoting child survival. 2010. Available: http://www.mchip.net/sites/default/files/USAID%20CBPHC%20FINAL.pdf. Accessed: 3 April 2017.

51 Jennings M, Pradhan S, Schleiff M, Sacks E, Freeman P, Gupta S, et al. Comprehensive review of the evidence regarding the effectiveness of community-based primary health care in improving maternal, neonatal and child health: 2. maternal health findings. J Glob Health. 2017;7:010902.

52 Sacks E, Freeman P, Sakyi K, Jennings M, Rassekh B, Gupta S, et al. Comprehensive review of the evidence regarding the effectiveness of community-based primary health care in improving maternal, neonatal and child health: 3. neonatal health findings. J Glob Health. 2017;7:010903.

53 Freeman P, Schleiff M, Sacks E, Rassekh B, Gupta S, Perry H. Comprehensive review of the evidence regarding the effectiveness of community-based primary health care in improving maternal, neonatal and child health: 4. child health findings. J Glob Health. 2017;7:010904.

54 Gwatkin DR, Wilcox JR, Wray JD. Can health and nutrition interventions make a difference? Washington, DC: Overseas Development Council; 1980.

55 Bryce J, Gilroy K, Jones G, Hazel E, Black RE, Victora CG. The Accelerated Child Survival and Development programme in west Africa: a retrospective evaluation. Lancet. 2010;375:572-82. Medline:20071020 doi:10.1016/S0140-6736(09)62060-2

56 Azad K, Barnett S, Banerjee B, Shaha S, Khan K, Rego AR, et al. Effect of scaling up women's groups on birth outcomes in three rural districts in Bangladesh: a cluster-randomised controlled trial. Lancet. 2010;375:1193-202. Medline:20207412 doi:10.1016/S0140-6736(10)60142-0

57 Evaluation: the top priority for global health. Lancet. 2010;375:526.

58 Perry H, Rassekh B, Gupta S, Freeman P. Comprehensive review of the evidence re-
    garding the effectiveness of community-based primary health care in improving ma-
    ternal, neonatal and child health: 7. shared characteristics of projects with evidence of
    long–term mortality impact. J Glob Health. 2017;7:010309.

59 McCord C, Chowdhury Q. A cost effective small hospital in Bangladesh: what it
    can mean for emergency obstetric care. Int J Gynaecol Obstet. 2003;81:83-92. Med-
    line:12676406 doi:10.1016/S0020-7292(03)00072-9

60 Gosselin RA, Thind A, Bellardinelli A. Cost/DALY averted in a small hospital in Sierra
    Leone: what is the relative contribution of different services? World J Surg. 2006;30:505-
    11. Medline:16528459 doi:10.1007/s00268-005-0609-5

61 Black RE, Levin C, Walker N, Chou D, Liu L, Temmerman M, et al. Reproductive,
    maternal, newborn, and child health: key messages from Disease Control Priorities
    3rd Edition. Lancet. 2016;388:2811-24.

62 Glenton C, Colvin CJ, Carlsen B, Swartz A, Lewin S, Noyes J, et al. Barriers and facili-
    tators to the implementation of lay health worker programmes to improve access to
    maternal and child health: qualitative evidence synthesis. Cochrane Database Syst Rev.
    2013;8:CD010414. Medline:24101553

63 Special Programme for Research and Training in Tropical Diseases. Community-direct-
    ed Interventions for Major Health Problems in Africa: A Final Multi-Country Report.
    Geneva, Switzerland: World Health Organization, 2008.

64 Marston C, Hinton R, Kean S, Baral S, Ahuja A, Costello A, et al. Community partici-
    pation for transformative action on women's, children's and adolescents' health. Bull
    World Health Organ. 2016;94:376-82. Medline:27152056 doi:10.2471/BLT.15.168492

65 WHO. The Global Strategy for Women's, Children's and Adolescents' Health (2016-
    2030): Survive, Thrive, Transform. 2016. Available: https://www.usaid.gov/sites/de-
    fault/files/Final-AOTC-file-v2.pdf. Accessed: 3 April 2017.

66 Curry DW, Perry HB, Tirmizi SN, Goldstein AL, Lynch MC. Assessing the effectiveness
    of house-to-house visits on routine oral polio immunization completion and tracking
    of defaulters. J Health Popul Nutr. 2014;32:356-66. Medline:25076672

67 Victora C. Presentation. Global Forum for Health Research; Mexico City2004.

68 Rifkin SB, Muller F, Bichmann W. Primary health care: on measuring participation. Soc
    Sci Med. 1988;26:931-40. Medline:3388072 doi:10.1016/0277-9536(88)90413-3

69 Molyneux S, Atela M, Angwenyi V, Goodman C. Community accountability at periph-
    eral health facilities: a review of the empirical literature and development of a con-
    ceptual framework. Health Policy Plan. 2012;27:541-54. Medline:22279082 doi:10.1093/
    heapol/czr083

70 Farmer P, Leandre F, Mukherjee JS, Claude M, Nevil P, Smith-Fawzi MC, et al. Commu-
    nity-based approaches to HIV treatment in resource-poor settings. Lancet. 2001;358:404-9.
    Medline:11502340 doi:10.1016/S0140-6736(01)05550-7

71 Chowdhury AM, Chowdhury S, Islam MN, Islam A, Vaughan JP. Control of tuber-
    culosis by community health workers in Bangladesh. Lancet. 1997;350:169-72. Med-
    line:9250184 doi:10.1016/S0140-6736(96)11311-8

72 Prata N, Vahidnia F, Potts M, Dries-Daffner I. Revisiting community-based distribu-
    tion programs: are they still needed? Contraception. 2005;72:402-7. Medline:16307960
    doi:10.1016/j.contraception.2005.06.059

73 Mishra SR, Neupane D, Preen D, Kallestrup P, Perry HB. Mitigation of non-communi-
    cable diseases in developing countries with community health workers. Global Health.
    2015;11:43. Medline:26555199 doi:10.1186/s12992-015-0129-5

Acknowledgement: *originally published as: Henry B Perry, Emma Sacks, Meike Schleiff, Richard Kumapley, Sundeep Gupta, Bahie M Rassekh, Paul A Freeman:Comprehensive review of the evidence regarding the effectiveness of Community–Based Primary Health Care in improving maternal, neonatal and child health: 6. strategies used by effective projects. Reprinted with permission from Edinburgh University Global Health Society under Creative Commons Attribution Licence (Journal of Global Health 2017; 010906).*

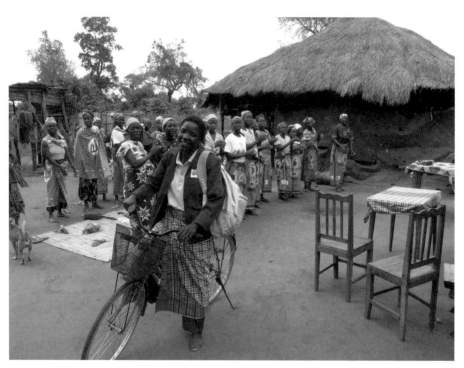

Photo credit: Tom Davis, MPH (used with permission).

Comprehensive review of the evidence regarding the effectiveness of community–based primary health care in improving maternal, neonatal and child health: 7. shared characteristics of projects with evidence of long–term mortality impact

Henry B Perry[1], Bahie M Rassekh[2], Sundeep Gupta[3], Paul A Freeman[4,5]

[1] Department of International Health, Johns Hopkins Bloomberg School of Public Health, Baltimore, Maryland, USA
[2] The World Bank, Washington, District of Columbia, USA
[3] Medical Epidemiologist, Lusaka, Zambia
[4] Independent consultant, Seattle, Washington, USA
[5] Department of Global Health, University of Washington, Seattle, Washington, USA

Background There is limited evidence about the long–term effectiveness of integrated community–based primary health care (CBPHC) in improving maternal, neonatal and child health. However, the interventions implemented and the approaches used by projects with such evidence can provide guidance for ending preventable child and maternal deaths by the year 2030.

Methods A database of 700 assessments of the effectiveness of CBPHC in improving maternal, neonatal and child health has been assembled, as described elsewhere in this series. A search was undertaken of these assessments of research studies, field project and programs (hereafter referred to as projects) with more than a single intervention that had evidence of mortality impact for a period of at least 10 years. Four projects qualified for this analysis: the Matlab Maternal Child Health and Family Planning (MCH–FP) Project in Bangladesh; the Hôpital Albert Schweitzer in Deschapelles, Haiti; the Comprehensive Rural Health Project (CRHP) in Jamkhed, India; and the Society for Education, Action and Research in Community Health (SEARCH) in Gadchiroli, India.

Results These four projects have all been operating for more than 30 years, and they all have demonstrated reductions in infant mortality, 1– to 4–year mortality, or under–5 mortality for at least 10 years. They share a number of characteristics. Among the most notable of these are: they provide comprehensive maternal, child health and family planning services, they have strong community–based programs that utilize community health workers who maintain regular contact with all households, they have develop strong collaborations with the communities they serve, and they all have strong referral capabilities and provide first–level hospital care.

Conclusions The shared features of these projects provide guidance for how health systems around the world might improve their effectiveness in improving maternal, neonatal and child health. Strengthening these features will contribute to achieving the goal of ending preventable child and maternal deaths by the year 2030.

Sustainability of effectiveness in improving maternal, neonatal and child health (MNCH) is an ideal that all MNCH programs seek. However, specially funded projects that undergo evaluation usually have a relatively short duration of five years or less. National demographic and health surveys may show long–term national improvements in child health, but determining the programmatic factors responsible for those improvements is difficult. As we have seen in this series of articles, the evidence regarding the effectiveness of community–based primary health care (CBPHC) in improving MNCH is based primarily on short–term assessments of a smaller group of selected interventions. Although two–thirds (66.7%) of the 152 maternal health assessments in our review were of projects with more than five interventions, only 15.8% of the projects were assessed for five or more years. Three–fourths of the 548 assessments of neonatal/child health projects included in our review assessed four or fewer interventions that were implemented over a period of less than five years.

However, one important question this review can address is: *What packages of community–based primary health care activities have produced evidence of long–term impact on MNCH?* A related question is: *Are there any common implementation strategies that these programs have in common that might help to explain their long–term effectiveness?* The answers to such questions can be helpful in considering how CBPHC can most effectively improve the health of mothers, neonates and children at scale over the longer term in high–mortality, resource–constrained settings.

The purpose of the current paper is to review the database assembled for the current journal supplement, of which this article is a part, and to describe the features of projects with more than one intervention that have evidence of long–term impact on maternal, neonatal or child health.

METHODS

The database of assessments of the effectiveness of CBPHC in improving MNCH has been described elsewhere in this series [1]. In short, it consists of data extracted from 700 documents describing the effectiveness of one or more interventions that have been implemented in the community outside of a health facility. Each assessment consisted of measurements of changes in maternal, neonatal and child health in terms of changes in population coverage of one or more evidence–based child survival interventions, in nutritional status, in serious morbidity, or in mortality. We queried this database for programs/projects/studies (hereafter referred to as projects) that had a duration of 10 years or more. Three assessments in the maternal health database were identified, and none of these met the criteria for this analysis. Twenty–one assessments in the neonatal/child health database were identified. Of these, 14 did not meet the criteria for this study for the reasons shown in **Figure 1**.

As shown in **Table 1**, 17 assessments of projects having a duration of 10 years or more were excluded from this analysis primarily because no measure of changes in mortality were available or the project implemented only one intervention.

The remaining seven assessments [2–8] that qualified for the analysis concerned four projects:
- The icddrb MCH–FP project in Matlab, Bangladesh;
- The Hôpital Albert Schweitzer in Deschapelles, Haiti (which operates a CBPHC program);

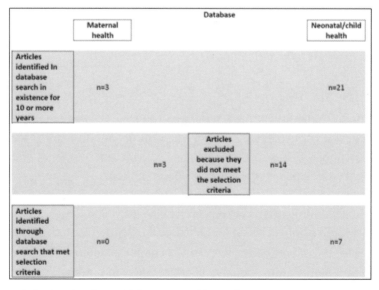

Figure 1. *Selection of projects with long-term evidence of impact on maternal or neonatal/child health through integrated community-based primary health care (CBPHC).*

Table 1. *Reasons for exclusion of assessments of projects of 10 or more years' duration*

REASON FOR EXCLUSION	PROJECTS OF 10-YEAR DURATION OR MORE EXCLUDED FROM ANALYSIS	
	Maternal database	Neonatal/child health database
No measure of mortality included	1	5
No baseline measure of mortality	2	2
Mortality impact data covered less than 10 years of programming		2
Only 1 intervention implemented		3*
No evidence or mortality impact		1
No comparison area		1
Total	3	14

*Vitamin A in one assessment, malaria control in one assessment, and conditional cash transfers in another assessment.

- The Jamkhed Comprehensive Health Project in Jamkhed, India; and,
- SEARCH (Society for Education, Action and Research in Community Health) in Gadchiroli, India.

Additional literature on these projects was reviewed, and additional findings were incorporated based on personal experience and field visits of one of the authors (HP) to these projects along with personal communications with persons engaged in these projects. By coincidence, Dr Perry worked in Bangladesh from 1995–1999 and visited the Matlab field site on a number of occasions. He served as Director General/CEO of the Hôpital Albert Schweitzer in Deschapelles, Haiti from 1999–2003. He has visited the CRHP project on four separate occasions (1998, 2004, 2006 and 2009) and the SEARCH project on two occasions (2004 and 2006).

RESULTS

The four projects identified from our database that had evidence of under–5 mortality impact for 10 years have each been functioning for 30 years or longer and are still functioning. These projects also had considerable evidence of improvements in coverage of key evidence–based interventions. These four projects are:

- The icddrb MCH–FP project in Matlab, Bangladesh (a maternal/child health and family planning research field site for icddrb, formerly known as the International Centre for Diarrhoeal Disease Research, Bangladesh);
- The Hôpital Albert Schweitzer in Deschapelles, Haiti;
- The Jamkhed Comprehensive Health Project in Jamkhed, India; and,
- SEARCH (Society for Education, Action and Research in Community Health) in Gadchiroli, India.

Here we describe below the main features of these projects, recognizing that over such a long period of time these features have not remained static. Nonetheless, the descriptions are appropriate for the time in which the mortality impacts were achieved even though they may not entirely accurately describe current activities.

The Icddrb MCH–FP project in Matlab (Bangladesh)

Project description

The Cholera Research Laboratory (CRL) was established in 1960 in Dhaka, Bangladesh to develop methods for preventing and treating cholera. In 1963, the CRL established a field site in a rural riverine area three hours southeast of Dhaka in a cholera–endemic area to test new approaches for controlling the disease, including the testing of the effectiveness of new cholera vaccines. In 1966, a Demographic Surveillance System (DSS) was established at Matlab with the initial goal of assessing the impact of new vaccines on morbidity and mortality. The DSS has become the oldest demographic surveillance system in the world, and Matlab is the site of hundreds of field research projects regarding health, nutrition, population and socio–economic development. The CRL expanded its work to maternal/child health and family planning in 1977, and in 1978 the Government of Bangladesh established the International Centre for Diarrheal Disease Research, Bangladesh (now icddrb), which took over responsibility for the Matlab DSS and field activities [9–11].

The field site is divided into two parts. The first is an Intervention Area, where intensified community–based health and family planning activities operated by icddrb began in 1977. This is the Maternal–Child Health and Family Planning (MCH–FP) project. The second is a Comparison Area, where only government health services are provided. Each of these two areas has a population of approximately 112 000 persons.

Eighty paid community health workers (CHWs) in the Intervention Area visit each home on a regular basis. (The frequency of visits has declined gradually from every two weeks in 1977 to every two months at present.) Each CHW is responsible for approximately 200 households and typically visits 20 homes per day. At the time of a home visit, the CHWs immunize women and children, provide antenatal and postnatal care, and treat childhood pneumonia according to WHO guidelines. They provide nutrition education and treat diarrheal disease. They also leave packs of oral rehydration salts (ORS) with a "depot holder," who is a mother in the neighborhood with additional training in the treatment of childhood diarrhea. Finally, the CHWs promote family planning, distribute birth control pills and condoms, administer injectable contraceptives and track pregnancies.

The CHWs working in the icddrb MCH–FP project are well–trained and well–supported, and they can refer patients to a nearby sub–center staffed by a full–time paramedic who provides routine maternal and child health care as well as reproductive health care. A hospital operated by the project is readily available for referrals. This referral system and readily available hospital care was a key element of the initial CRL activity since the survival of patients with cholera depended on prompt identification and transport, usually by boat in this riverine environment, to the hospital in Matlab operated by the CRL. The project earned a high level of trust with the population because of the high quality of health care it has provided over four decades. Maintaining good relations with the community is a priority for the Matlab MCH–FP project, and project managers promptly address any issues raised by the community about the quality of services or the nature of the field research activities. The total annual cost per capita for the community–based portion of the health project (excluding research–related expenses) is about US$ 5 [12].

Four sub–centers are located in the Intervention Area (one for about 28 000 people), and 20 CHWs are assigned to each sub–center, where a full–time paramedic works. CHWs meet at the sub–center every two weeks for supervision, continuing education, and replenishment of supplies. Basic comprehensive primary health care is provided by the paramedics, including insertion of IUDs, menstrual regulation (suction curettage of the uterus for women with delayed menstrual periods who do not want to become pregnant), and treatment of sexually transmitted diseases and reproductive tract infections. Icddrb also operates a 50–bed inpatient facility that serves the Intervention Area. A government district hospital serving a larger geographic area is also in Matlab. Major surgical procedures are not available at the icddrb Matlab facility, but emergency obstetrical care, including caesarian section, is provided in collaboration with the government district hospital in Matlab [12].

Key components for success at Matlab include:
- Sound organizational structure from the outset;
- Readily available transport throughout the project area, mostly by speedboat, which has facilitated patient referral to the Matlab Hospital;
- A strong system of accompaniment and support for all levels of workers;
- A well–developed record–keeping system; and
- Continuously available supplies.

The book *Matlab: Women, Children and Health* provides a full discussion of the history of Matlab, its operations and research findings through the early 1990s [10].

Long–term outcomes

In 1984, the contraceptive prevalence rate (CPR) in the Intervention Area was 46% compared while it was 16% in the Comparison Area and 19% nationwide. In 2005, the CPR in the Intervention Area was 71%, 47% in the Comparison Area, and 58% nationwide. In 1987, the coverage rate for the standard series of childhood immunizations was 69% in the Intervention Area compared to a national rate of approximately 20% nationwide [12]. In 2005, the childhood immunization coverage rate in the Intervention Area was 97% compared to 85% in the Comparison Area.

Between 1988 and 1993, the mortality rate from pneumonia in children younger than 2 years of age was 54% lower in the Intervention Area than in the Comparison Area [13]. There was a reduction by around 75% in the annual number of childhood deaths over a 25–year period in Matlab, and over a 40-year–period, life expectancy increased from 50 to around 65 years [10].

The infant and 1– to 4–year mortality rates for the Intervention Area of MCH–FP project area were consistently lower than in the government services area (the Control Area) over a 15–year period between 1978 and 1994 [14,15]. In 1985, the under–five mortality rate (U5MR) per 1000 live births was approximately 200 in the Comparison Area and 150 in the Intervention Area (25% less). In 1995, the rates were approximately 120 and 75 respectively (38% less in the Intervention Area). In 2005, the under–five mortality rate was 46.6 in the intervention area and 62.4 in the Comparison Area (25% less) [14,15]. Over the period from 1982 to 2005, the maternal mortality rate (that is, the number of maternal deaths per 100 000 women of reproductive age) was 37% lower in the Intervention Area than in the Comparison Area, mainly as a result of a lower pregnancy rate and lower case–fatality rates for induced abortion, miscarriages and stillbirths [16].

The total fertility rate (TFR) over time has been the following: in 1985, the TFRs were 4.5 in the Intervention Area and 6.0 in the Comparison Area; in 1995, they were 3.0 and 3.6 respectively; by 2005, the rates were essentially the same at 2.7 and 2.8, respectively [14,15].

The progress in the Control Area can be attributed in part to the national application of the Matlab family planning model of home visits by paid workers to promote the use of family planning and the distribution of birth control pills and condoms. By the mid–1980s, Bangladesh essentially had a national CHW program. Progress in increasing the use of facilities for giving birth was slower in the Comparison Area. In 2004, only 12% of the births in the Comparison Area were taking place in a facility while in the Intervention Area the corresponding figure was 50% [14,15].

Lessons learned

Two lessons learned at Matlab and reported in 1994 bear emphasis here:

- "Family planning field workers are more likely to gain the confidence of the community if they respond to other health problems, particularly those of women and children.... [T]he benefits of integrating quality health services into a family planning programme justify the heavy inputs" [17].
- "The successful operation of such a large and multifaceted project as Matlab requires a professional level of organization in the hands of a competent manager. This applies for staff management, logistics and supplies, and relations with the community" [17].

One of the striking findings from the Matlab example is how quickly child mortality in the Comparison Area declined and how the difference between the Intervention and Comparison Areas gradually narrowed later. The differences in mortality rates for infants and children between the Intervention and Comparison Areas have narrowed over time. This can partly be explained by the fact that the MCH–FP Project at Matlab served as a model of CBPHC for the country, and Bangladesh has done a masterful job of extending home–based services – both MCH and FP services – throughout the country. Bangladesh is one of only 19 out of 68 high–mortality countries that reached the Millennium Development Goal for children by 2015 [18], and its national achievements in expanding coverage of community–based services has been widely documented and applauded [19]. After the interventions of the Matlab MCH–FP Project were proven to be effective in the 1970s, there was an explicit effort in the 1980s to introduce this same strategy nationally, with obvious benefits.

Hôpital Albert Schweitzer (Deschapelles, Haiti)

Project description

L'Hôpital Albert Schweitzer (HAS) began operations in 1956 after a wealthy American couple, William Larimer and Gwen Grant Mellon, were inspired by the example of the great medical missionary Albert Schweitzer who, for more than a half–century, provided medical care in Gabon, an underserved country of West Africa. The Mellons constructed one of Haiti's first modern hospitals in the Artibonite Valley, three hours northwest of capital, Port–au–Prince [20].

For the first decade of its existence, HAS provided only hospital care and services at an outpatient clinic based at the 190–bed hospital. In its second decade (in 1967), it established a project of community–based primary health care based on community health workers (*agents de santé*) and mobile health teams without any peripheral primary health care facilities. Over time, seven health posts and two health centers opened. The hospital always served as the Ministry of Health's district hospital for the health district in which it is located, with 258 000 people in its catchment area during most of the period covered by the impact assessment. The population served by HAS's primary health care project fluctuated over the years, from 18 820 in 1958 to 180 000 in 1996 and to 350 000 in 2016 [3,20].

In the 1960s, HAS also established community development activities, including projects for improving water and sanitation at the village and household levels, promoting vegetable gardens and reforestation, providing opportunities for micro–credit and income–generation for women, literacy training, support for primary education, and promotion of animal husbandry and improved agricultural production. HAS thus became a comprehensive integrated health and development system with strong CBPHC services together with facility–based primary health care, hospital referral care and community development activities [3].

The CBPHC services at HAS have relied on paid Health Agents (*Agents de Sante*) who regularly visit every home to provide basic health education, register vital events, and mobilize mothers and children to attend Rally Posts where essential services are provided, including immunizations, growth monitoring/promotion, and referral care at the hospital. Mobile clinics reach all isolated areas intermittently. These are staffed by an auxiliary nurse who, every 1–2 months, visits isolated communities on foot (since there are few roads in the mountains) to provide basic curative and preventive care (including family planning) and to refer patients when needed.

In the late 1990s, 1500 volunteer community health workers (*Animatrices*), one for every 15 households, were recruited to provide peer–to–peer health education to other women, to assist with the Rally Posts and Mobile Clinics, to promote community involvement, and to assist with referral of patients to higher levels of care [3]. In addition, eight Monitors (*Monitrices*) provide liaison with and training of lay midwives, along with supervising and training the *Animatrices*. The role of *Monitrices* at HAS initially involved supervising the community–based nutritional rehabilitation project, known as the Hearth Project, which originated at HAS and has been implemented in numerous other countries. Finally, the CBPHC services at HAS include 16 community–based tuberculosis workers (seven *Accompagnateurs* and nine *Agents*) who obtain sputum specimens from symptomatic patients and provide directly observed therapy for patients in their home. Community–based provision of anti–retroviral medication for patients with HIV/AIDS is now provided as well.

Steady financial support from external donors has been available to HAS since its inception, and this has helped HAS to provide high–quality professional leadership and management. It has been able to ensure logistical support for its field projects and to provide needed supplies and drugs. The quality of its clinical services has earned the trust and support of the population over a long period of time. The hospital is widely regarded as one of the best district hospitals in a rural area of a developing country, and patients from throughout Haiti have come there for treatment.

Long–term outcomes

In 2000, population coverage rates of key child survival interventions in the HAS primary health care service area were approximately twice those for the same interventions nationwide in rural Haiti. Additionally, the U5MR in the HAS service area was less than half of that for Haiti overall (62.3 vs 149.4) [3]. Likewise at that time, the CPR in the HAS project area was nearly double that in other areas (27.5% vs 15.4%) [3]. Great efforts have been made to ensure access to basic services in the most isolated parts of the HAS project area, some of which require eight–hours by foot to reach.

As a result of the collection of vital events data at the time of initiation of HAS's community health project in 1967 [21] and the intermittent collection of retrospective birth histories since, it has been possible to monitor the U5MR for the primary health care project area served by HAS and to compare these to data for Haiti as a whole. The HAS project area is similar in socio–economic indicators to rural Haiti as a whole [4].

The U5MR in the HAS primary health care service area remained much lower than in Haiti nationally over a three–decade period from 1970 to 1999 [4]. The rapid decline in under–five mortality to one–quarter of the national level between 1958 and 1973 was due in large part to the elimination of neonatal tetanus through immunization of all women of reproductive age [22,23]. Between 1970 and 1999, the U5MR remained less than half that of the U5MR for Haiti [4].

The per capita annual cost for the entire project as it existed in 1999 would be US$ 24.77 in 2016 dollars. Because of resource constraints, the projects at HAS have undergone significant cutbacks over the past decade. The cost per under–five death averted in current dollars was US$ 3233; the cost per year of live saved was US$ 47; and the cost per DALY saved was US$ 90 [24].

Lessons learned

There does not appear to be any single intervention or even a small set of interventions responsible for the sustained mortality reduction. Rather, the entire system of health and development – community–based services, primary health care services at health posts and health centers, hospital services, community development projects, as well as the interactions between these elements – most likely contributed to this mortality impact. The close integration of the CBPHC activities with the primary health care facilities and the hospital are key elements of system effectiveness.

The rapid decline of mortality for Haiti as a whole during the period from 1970–1999, is worth noting, particularly in light of the country's political instability, its deteriorating economic situation, and the epidemic of HIV/AIDS throughout the country, which began in the early 1980s. In fact, in spite of the devastating earthquake in the capital in 2010 and more recent cholera outbreaks, Haiti is one of only 34 of the 74 so–called Countdown Countries (with 97% of world's maternal and child deaths) to have achieved the Millennium Development Goals in 2015 for reduction in child and maternal mortality [25]. The model of CBPHC developed at HAS is now utilized by virtually all other NGOs working in community health in the country, and these NGOs provide community–based child survival services to two–thirds of the population of Haiti. The nationwide contribution of CBPHC to the gains achieved in child survival in Haiti have been possible in part because of the early experience at HAS and its position as a role model for the rest of the country.

India: the Jamkhed Comprehensive Rural Health Project

Project description

The Jamkhed Comprehensive Rural Health Project (CRHP) in Ahmednagar District of Maharashtra, India, has been in operation for almost five decades [5,26]. It developed a comprehensive approach to community–based health programming in conjunction with first–level hospital referral services. Its principles of equity, integration and empowerment have been guiding principles throughout this prolonged period.

When CRHP began in 1970, the people of the Jamkhed area were living in near–famine conditions from drought and lack of access to water. The prevalence of childhood malnutrition was 40%, and coverage rates of childhood immunizations, family planning, prenatal care, and birth attendance by a trained provider were all less than 1%; and the infant mortality rate was 176 per 1000 live births. The caste system was ingrained, and harmful traditional practices, especially for women, were common. In addition, women had no personal rights. Furthermore, they were often treated inhumanely. One–third of the population was migrating to sugar cane plantations outside of the district to work in temporary jobs because of the scarcity of food and the lack of work in the Jamkhed area.

Rajanikant and Mabelle Arole started working in Jamkhed in 1970 as a husband–wife physician team treating patients who came to them with medical problems. They quickly realized that over three–quarters of health problems could be addressed at the community level, mainly by the villagers themselves, if they had a modest amount of additional knowledge and skills. The main purpose of their work soon became to facilitate a process whereby communities could improve their health through their active participation by learning about and addressing their problems based on their own priorities.

Some of the initial activities carried out were: health promotion through health education, immunization, prenatal care, complementary infant feeding, ensuring safe delivery, family planning, and a health center for curative care. Their work gradually expanded to train illiterate CHWs, address the determinants of ill–health through improving access to water and food, nutrition education and kitchen gardens, women's and community empowerment, micro–credit, education, improved agriculture, and prioritizing the needs of the poorest and most disenfranchised members of communities. From the beginning, CRHP worked only with communities that requested assistance and committed themselves to participation. Gradually, all villages in the area sought to be involved as they saw the benefits to other communities from participation.

CRHP always insists on major investments of time and energy from community members as a condition of CRHP's entering into partnership with a community, so the process that emerged ensures future sustainability. The project established groups of volunteers within the community, including village health workers (VHWs), farmers' clubs and women's groups (*mahila mandals*), and, more recently, girls' and adolescent boys' groups.

The key change agent in the community became the VHW, who is selected by the community. She is eager to assist her village, especially the poorest and most marginalized members such as *Dalits* (untouchables) and those with stigmatized conditions (such as leprosy). She receives training in health, community development, communication, organization and personal development. Her primary role is to share her knowledge with everyone in the community, to organize community groups, and to facilitate the community's assessment of problems and resources, analysis of causes and determinants, and appropriate actions, especially with the poor and marginalized that might be undertaken with the assistance of CRHP. Initially, many of these VHWs were illiterate women from the untouchable (*dalit*) caste who had recovered from an illness (such as tuberculosis) as a result of care provided by CRHP.

Although the VHWs do not work for pay, with project assistance they obtain access to income–generating activities. They serve as a link between the community and the project's mobile team, which visits each village once a month or more often if needed. The mobile team consists of a nurse, an agricultural specialist and a social worker, though they all become multipurpose workers through working together, learning from each other, and additional training.

The VHWs come to the project center in the small town of Jamkhed once a week. There they meet with the other VHWs to discuss problems encountered in their work and to obtain further training from each other and from staff. They spend the night there and provide social support for each other. Many of the VHWs have been working for more than 30 years. Dropouts are rare, mainly because of old age and death.

For many years, CRHP operated a 30–bed hospital that served as a referral source for patients from the project area and beyond. A larger 50–bed hospital has recently been completed. Emergency cesarean section and other emergency surgical procedures are performed there. At the beginning of the project, the hospital in Jamkhed was filled with children who had life–threatening infections and malnutrition. Such patients are rarely seen there now.

CRHP gradually expanded to reach 300 villages with a population of 500 000 people. Most of these villages are now independent, thanks to the sustainable development process that CRHP has nurtured over five decades, so CRHP now focuses on the villages that need them most.

Because of the great interest of people throughout India and the world to learn about the CRHP experience, the Jamkhed International Institute for Training and Research in Community Health and Development was established in 1992. More than 30 000 people from throughout India and more than 3000 people from over 100 countries have come there to learn from the VHWs, other villagers and CRHP staff and to visit villages to see the impact firsthand.

Each village maintains a record of all births and deaths that take place among its members, as well as records of the number of eligible couples who are using family planning, the number of children completely immunized, and the number of children with malnutrition. Also included is information about socioeconomic conditions, agricultural and environmental issues, and various priority diseases. This information is written on a board that is displayed in a public space in the village and services as a focal point for discussions about priorities for the community to address. Participatory Rural Appraisal (PRA) techniques are commonly used for assessments and analysis as well as for discussions on what to do. All segments of the community participate.

Long–term outcomes

By 1993, the percentage of pregnant women with antenatal care and a safe delivery reached 82% and, in 2011, it reached 99%. The percentage of couples utilizing family planning reached 68% in 2004. In 2004, 87% of children were fully immunized and only 5% were undernourished according to anthropometric measurements. This low prevalence of undernutrition has been maintained ever since. Leprosy, which was common at the start of the project, has virtually disappeared, and the incidence of tuberculosis has declined from 1800 to 200 cases per 100 000 persons [26].

The IMR at CRHP Jamkhed declined from 176 deaths per 1000 live births in 1971 to 19 in 1993 [5] to 8 in 2011, according to data collected at CRHP by CHWs [26]. In 1971, the IMR at CRHP Jamkhed was 60% greater than for the rural area of the state of Maharashtra (176 vs 110), but since 1980 the IMR at CRHP Jamkhed has been half that for rural Maharashtra [27]. A large–scale external and independent evaluation of the mortality impact of CRHP based on a comparison of findings from birth histories in project villages with those in a surrounding control area was carried out in 2007–8. This evaluation demonstrated a 30% reduction in the risk of death among children 1–59 months of age in CRHP project villages compared to control villages [28].

Although baseline levels of maternal and perinatal mortality were not measured in the 1970s when CRHP began, these rates were measured following a careful review of all births and deaths in 25 villages around Jamkhed between 1996 and 1999. A maternal mortality ratio of 70.0 per 100 000 live births and a perinatal mortality rate of 36.0 per 1000 live births and stillbirths were measured at CRHP [29]. These rates were 27.8% and 20.3% lower respectively than the maternal and perinatal mortality for Pune district in Maharashtra State in India, were the CRHP is located [29].

These significant results were accomplished because of the communities' participation and empowerment together with their understanding of health promotion and disease prevention. For example, family members know the importance of healthy nutritional practices, prenatal care, how to provide early home care for common problems (such as homemade oral rehydration solution for diarrhea, steam inhalation for respiratory problems, sponging with cool water for fever, and sunlight for neonatal jaundice). VHWs ensure exclusive breastfeeding for infants during their first 6 months of life, proper burping after feeding, and nutritional weaning foods. The men and women's groups weigh the children for growth monitoring. Immunizations were also gradually accepted by the communities as the program developed. The government now provides these services with the support and cooperation of the VHWs and community groups.

In the early years the communities organized feeding programs for groups of children, with everyone contributing something (eg, firewood, water, salt, grains, or pulses), and the Farmers' Clubs dedicated some of their land for growing food for the program. They established watershed development projects to increase the available of groundwater for home and agricultural use. Most homes now have kitchen gardens for additional, nutritious fruits and vegetables.

Lessons learned

To be sure, the impact of CRHP is demonstrated through changes in health statistics, which show positive results achieved over more than four decades. Behind these statistics are self–confident men and women, once outside the mainstream of society, taking leadership positions in their villages, affirming that they have God–given dignity, worth and capacity. Thus, it is not only the quantitative changes that are important. Even more important is the transfor-mation of persons and communities in a qualitative way, which have made these health improvements possible.

Community empowerment increases self–reliance, self–esteem, self–confi-dence – and it reduces dependency on outside agencies. In order for the de-velopment process to be sustainable by the people, the community must have good leadership and the capacity to address its own issues. In the Jamkhed process, the community learns to work together and solve problems together. If the community needs more knowledge, skills or resources, CRHP helps them.

The Jamkhed process of sustained health improvement through CBPHC in-volves:

- Expanding knowledge and skills through building the capabilities of in-dividuals and communities, based on where they are and what they have.
- Developing a caring and sharing community that promotes reconcilia-tion and peace (*shalom*) by engaging the whole community, including the poorest and most marginalized members and integrating them as active members of the community to solve the problems that concern them most through assessment, analysis, and action.
- Promoting volunteerism by building a community of motivated and caring individuals committed to engaging in these activities.
- Focusing on low–cost activities including home remedies and herbal medicines as well as health promotion, prevention, early detection, treat-ment, and rehabilitation in the community.
- Utilizing appropriate technology and local resources that are accessible in the context of the community's knowledge, skills and interests.

- Engaging in multi–sectoral development, including education, sanitation and income generation, as well as building social capital and helping people to recognize the harm that some traditional practices are causing for the purpose of improving the overall well–being of the community, recognizing that conditions outside of the health sector have more impact on health than curative care alone.
- Recruiting, training and supporting women VHWs, who are so motivated that after decades of service they are still active leaders, still learning and sharing with their communities and others.

This transformative process is spread to other communities by the villagers who have experienced it, making it a people's movement. This is not an innovation in technology but rather an innovation from within each community that brings about social change and thereby uplifts everyone from poverty and disease. Lives are transformed by embracing the dignity and worth of everyone and giving an opportunity to all to contribute.

CRHP is one of the world's leading examples of improving MNCH through community empowerment, women's empowerment and community partici- pation. In spite of not being well–known in academic and research circles, it is well known in the broader global health community through the visits of thousands of people from throughout India and around the world as well as through the 1994 publication of the acclaimed book by the Aroles, simply entitled *Jamkhed: A Comprehensive Rural Health Project* [5]. This book is one of the best long–term sellers among global health books and has been translated into a number of different languages.

Of historical importance is the fact that the CRHP served as one of the in- spirations for the 1978 International Conference on Primary Health Care at Alma–Ata. CRHP was one of the projects featured in the influential monograph published by the World Health Organization several years prior to the Con- ference [30,31]. In contrast to the limited information in most peer–reviewed scientific articles regarding the context within which CBPHC operates and how it is actually implemented in the community, there is extensive information about these benchmarks in the acclaimed book by the Aroles [5].

SEARCH (Society for Education, Action and Research in Community Health) in Gadchiroli, India

Project description

Since 1986, the Society for Education, Action, and Research in Community Health (SEARCH) has provided community–based health care services and hospital care in a rural area of the state of Maharashtra, India, known as Gadchiroli [32,33]. The Gadchiroli District is the least developed in the state. The district is largely forested, and half of the inhabitants are indigenous tribal people who live in the forest. The other half is composed predominantly of Hindu subsistence farmers. Gadchiroli is 175 km south of Nagpur in the most western part of Maharashtra.

The founders, Dr Abhay Bang and Dr Rani Bang, were inspired by the life of Mahatma Gandhi and established their work in the context of Gandhian social philosophy. They developed a collaborative partnership with the communities of Gadchiroli for basic health care, education and training in health, and for research to inform health policies [34]. Like the Aroles, who founded the Jamkhed CRHP Project, the Bangs obtained important insights for their work from the Narangwal Project, a model community health project established in collaboration with the Johns Hopkins University in the 1970s [35,36].

The Bangs established three goals for their organization: (1) provide health care to the local population, (2) provide training and education in health, and (3) conduct research to shape health policies. The vision of SEARCH is the realization of *Aarogya–Swaraj* (translated as "the people's health in people's hands") by empowering individuals and communities to take charge of their own health, thereby helping them achieve freedom from disease as well as from dependence. The mission of SEARCH is expressed in its name, "Society for Education, Action and Research in Community Health." The mission is "to work with marginalized communities to identify their health needs, develop community–empowering models of health care to meet these health needs, to test these models by way of research studies, and then to make this knowledge available to others by way of training and publications" [32]. Thus, community–based primary health care, community participatory research and training of village people are core activities at SEARCH.

Over the past 30 years, Drs. Abhay and Rani Bang and their dedicated staff developed a community health project that provides community–based primary health care for a population of 80 000 people. One–half of this area is used as a field site for implementing new interventions while the other half serves as a control area in the sense that the new intervention is not being implemented there during the study period. SEARCH also operates a 20–bed hospital and outpatient facility to serve tribal people from the area.

SEARCH pioneered the development of a community–based reproductive health care project and related research. It also developed a pioneering community collaboration to address alcohol and drug addiction, which was initiated in response to requests from the community [37]. Basic surgical services are provided at the hospital, including cesarean sections and surgical care for a common cause of long–term disability – massive hydrocele caused by lymphatic filariasis. Patients requiring higher levels of care are transported to a government hospital in the city of Gadchiroli, which is about 30 minutes away. The staff at SEARCH consists of 30 members, including physicians, paramedics, project supervisors and managers, and research staff.

SEARCH established a partnership with communities over the past two decades by listening to members, responding to their expressed concerns and priorities, and involving them in the planning, implementation and evaluation of its projects. The community has taken co–ownership of the project.

SEARCH does not duplicate the government health system. Instead, it has developed a community–based health provision system that utilizes the government health system for referrals. SEARCH employs, trains and supervises one female community health worker (CHW) for approximately every 1000 population. This CHW visits every home on a monthly basis, registers pregnancies, births and deaths since the previous visit, and provides health education and basic preventive and curative health care. By maintaining close contact with the households for which she is responsible, the CHW is able to provide childhood pneumonia treatment and home–based neonatal care along with other basic health care services for mothers and children. Between 1988 and 2005, SEARCH also provided strong training and support for the traditional village midwives (*dais*).

The Bang's groundbreaking research on the effectiveness of community–case management of childhood pneumonia [38] and on the effectiveness of home–based neonatal care [2] has had a major impact on health care programs throughout the developing world. The project relies on trained traditional birth attendants and community health workers for diagnosis and treatment of common illnesses, diagnosis and treatment of childhood pneumonia, and provision of home–based neonatal care.

Long–term outcomes

The infant mortality rate in the Intervention Area declined by 74%, from 120 deaths per 1000 live births in 1988 to 31 in 2003 [2,39]. In the Comparison Area, over the period of time for which data have been reported (1994–2004), the IMR remained essentially unchanged [2,39]. This was the period during which the home–based neonatal care intervention was being implemented and evaluated.

Lessons learned

The pioneering findings of the community case management of pneumonia and of home–based neonatal care by SEARCH in Gadchiroli have stimulated much additional work by others around the world since the efficacy of these interventions were first reported by the Bangs in the 1990s [38,40]. The Bangs provided leadership for replication of the home–based neonatal care intervention by other NGOs in the state of Maharashtra, and they provided technical assistance for scaled–up versions of the SEARCH model for home–based neonatal care now being tested by the India Council of Medical Research at various sites around India.

Among other things, their work has demonstrated that properly trained, supervised and supported CHWs, even if they are illiterate, can provide high–quality technical interventions for mothers and children. The methods of selection, training and support of CHWs used by SEARCH merit closer analysis and widespread application.

DISCUSSION

The Matlab MCH–FP project in rural Bangladesh, the HAS integrated project of health and development in rural Haiti, the Jamkhed CRHP in rural India, and the Gadchiroli SEARCH project in rural India are among the few examples that exist of projects with evidence of long-term reductions in maternal, neonatal or child mortality resulting from community–based interventions. Three of the four of these projects have been in operation for more than four decades, while the fourth (SEARCH) has been in operation for more than three decades.

Common characteristics of projects with evidence of long–term impact on mortality

What is particularly striking is the similarity of many of the features of these projects. As **Table 2** demonstrates, all four of these projects are similar in the broad range of services they offer along the continuum of care for individuals at various points in the life cycle – from pregnancy and childbirth to the neonatal and child periods to adolescent and adulthood. They are also similar in the breadth of types of services – from preventive to curative to rehabilitative services. Finally, they are similar in the vertical integration of their services – from home–based and community–based services all the way to hospital referral services.

Table 2. *Common characteristics of four projects with long–term evidence of impact on child mortality**

Characteristic	Hôpital Albert Schweitzer (Haiti)	Matlab MCH–FP project (Bangladesh)	CRHP– Jamkhed (India)	SEARCH– Gadchiroli (India)
Basic project characteristics:				
Year established	1956	1965	1970	1986
Population of catchment area	150 000	100 000	300 000	80 000†
Range of services provided:				
Is a comprehensive array of child health services provided? These include health and nutrition education, diagnosis and treatment of acute childhood illness, referral of seriously ill children to a higher level of care.	Yes	Yes	Yes	Yes
Is a comprehensive array of maternal, reproductive health, and family planning services provided? These include health and nutrition education, provision of antenatal care, management and/or referral of obstetrical complications, provision of postnatal care, and provision of a wide range of family planning methods	Yes	Yes	Yes	Yes
Are general curative services provided? These include treatment of common childhood illnesses and management (including referral when indicated) of serious childhood illnesses in the community; care for acute illnesses among patients of all ages in health centers, and referral of seriously ill patients to higher levels of care.	Yes	Yes	Yes	Yes
Are surgical and/or other hospital inpatient services provided?	Yes (operates its own first–level referral hospital with advanced surgical capabilities)	Yes (operates its own first–level referral hospital with no surgical capabilities)	Yes (operates its own first–level referral hospital with advanced surgical capabilities)	Yes (operates its own first–level referral hospital with some surgical capabilities, eg, cesarean section)
How strong is the referral system from the community to higher levels of care at fixed facilities, including hospitals? In all four projects, a first–level referral hospital is integrated into the project. However, all surgical cases at Matlab are referred to the government district hospital as are more complicated surgical cases at Jamkhed and SEARCH.	Very strong	Very strong	Very strong	Very strong

Table 2. *Continued*

CHARACTERISTIC	HÔPITAL ALBERT SCHWEITZER (HAITI)	MATLAB MCH–FP PROJECT (BANGLADESH)	CRHP– JAMKHED (INDIA)	SEARCH– GADCHIRO- LI (INDIA)
Health project management and support:				
Does the project have a strong system of management and supervision led by competent and dedicated profes- sionals?	Yes	Yes	Yes	Yes
Does the project have a record of ac- complishment in treating patients and clients with a high level of respect?	Yes	Yes	Yes	Yes
Does the project have a record of main- taining supplies and drugs?	Yes	Yes	Yes	Yes
Nature of community partnerships/ community involvement:				
How strong is the partnership be- tween the project and the community?	Fairly strong	Fairly strong	Very strong	Very strong
How strong is the level of trust of the community in the project?	Very strong	Very strong	Very strong	Very strong
Role of community–based workers:				
Are CHWs an integral part of the project?	Yes	Yes	Yes	Yes
Do CHWs receive financial support?	Yes	Yes	Yes‡	Yes
How strong is the training and sup- port of CHWs?	Very strong	Very strong	Very strong	Very strong
Do CHWs have routine contact with all families through visitation of all homes?	Yes	Yes	Yes§	Yes
Do CHWs provide essential child health services in the home?	Yes	Yes	Yes	Yes

CHW – community health worker

*Some of this information is based on the authors' field observations and discussions with project leaders and is not contained in written documents.

†The part of the SEARCH project area with documented declines in infant mortality has 40 000 people.

‡Although the CRHP CHWs do not receive a salary, they do receive special training and access to credit to enable them to become economically self–sufficient through their own income–generating activities. CRHP ensures that their CHWs have enough income to meet their needs.

Another characteristic these projects have in common is that they all have a strong community–oriented health system in which the community is a part- ner. Improving MNCH is one of many goals of the health system that these projects developed. However, they all also provide comprehensive primary health care services with a strong focus on maternal and reproductive health and family planning. They all provide hospital services and ensure that basic surgical care is available to the populations they serve. They all recognize the importance of a functioning referral system to ensure that patients can access higher levels of care when needed. Most importantly, all four of these integrated comprehensive projects have established strong CBPHC services that serve as a foundation upon which the other project activities rest. These CBPHC services all include strong collaborations and partnerships with communities.

All projects have strong professional leadership as well as dynamic management and supervisory systems. They ensure that essential supplies and drugs are available. They all have a record of treating patients with a high level of respect.

The projects have been developed and sustained with a high level of community engagement; the community has a high level of trust in the health services provided by the projects. The provision of a broad array of high–quality curative services by each of these projects over a long period of time has resulted in trust being developed with the communities.

A final important similarity is that all four projects created strong roles for community–level workers. The projects all realized their effectiveness would be compromised without building a central role for these workers, all of whom receive some type of financial assistance. These CHWs all receive high–quality training and supervisory support. They maintain routine contact with all families in service areas, and they provide essential health care in their homes and at readily accessible sites in the community and nearby.

These four projects have all influenced thinking and practice in CBPHC programming for MNCH around the world – through their research as well as through their influence on younger people who have had personal experiences in the field with these projects who later become global health leaders. And, of course, CRHP's influence on the emergence of primary health care as defined at Alma–Ata as well as on the later emergence of national CHW programs in India is well–known [31,41].

The findings reported in this paper have focused on long–term improvements in neonatal and child health. But, it is important to point out that two of the four projects included here also have evidence of long–term reductions in maternal mortality: Matlab MCH–FP [10] and CRHP [29]. Exploring these findings in detail is beyond the scope of this article, but suffice it to say here that presence of strong CBPHC interventions for reproductive and maternal health (including family planning) linked to well–developed referral systems and readily available hospital care serve as the foundation for preventing maternal deaths.

Another interesting shared characteristic is that each of the four projects has a "culture" of science and evaluation, which led to the reporting of outcomes and the inclusion of these four projects in our review. These projects have been at the forefront of generation of knowledge about effective programming based on their field experiences.

A final shared feature of these four projects is their strong connection to the Narangwal Project and Dr Carl Taylor. We noted previously that both CRHP and SEARCH were directly influenced by the Narangwal Project, a pioneering field project in north India during the late 1960s and early 1970s that was one of the first to carefully evaluate the effectiveness of community–based primary health care [26,35]. The Aroles and the Bangs were master of public health students of Dr Carl Taylor's at the Johns Hopkins University, where they learned about the Narangwal Project. The CBPHC work at icddrb was directly influence by the Narangwal Project as well because the director of fieldwork for that project, Dr Shusham Bhutyia, later initiated the training and support of CHWs for the Matlab MCH–FP project. The CBPHC work at HAS in Haiti was led by Drs. Warren and Gretchen Berggren, who were mentored in this by Dr John Wyon, a colleague of Dr Carl Taylor's in north India and the field director for the Khanna Study [42], a community–based field research project that served as a predecessor of the Narangwal Project. Dr Carl Taylor served as a mentor to John Wyon during the development and implementation of the Khanna Study and they remained close colleagues subsequently.

However, in spite of these many shared characteristics, there are important differences to note as well. There are notable differences in the four projects in terms of the degree to which they have engaged in research and reported their results in peer–reviewed journals. The Matlab MCH–FP project is one of the world's foremost field research sites. SEARCH has been the site of some of the most influential research in global health related to community–case management of pneumonia and home–based neonatal care. Although HAS and CRHP have been the site of important research, these two projects have had less of a research orientation and more of a service orientation.

The Matlab MCH–FP project differs importantly from the other three in that it functions within the strong institutional framework of an international research center without an obvious single strong small set of long–term leaders. The projects each had two key individuals who led them from the beginning over a long period of time. CRHP is notable compared to the others in its deep commitment to field–based education of thousands of people from around India and beyond who have come to learn about CRHP's approach to working with communities and CHWs.

Criticisms have commonly been made of smaller "model" CBPHC projects because (i) they are not sustainable and not scalable since they are dependent on charismatic leadership and (ii) they have not had to deal with the management and logistical challenges of operating a program at larger scale, which are an order of magnitude more difficult. From the standpoint of these four projects, it is obvious that they are sustainable because of their long–term operation. None of these projects attempted to go to scale, but in every case certain elements of each project have in fact been scaled up in an indirect sense. The Matlab MCH–FP Project, once proven effective, served as the model of government national scale up of CHW programming. HAS's approach to CHWs has been adopted by virtually all other NGOs providing community–based services throughout Haiti. The CRHP approach to CHWs has served as a model for national CHW programming in India, both with the Village Health Guides program of the 1980s and the more recently established ASHA program. SEARCH's demonstration of the effectiveness of community–based management of pneumonia and of home–based neonatal care interventions stimulated further independent confirmatory research. Now, this approach has become the global standard of care around the world in resource–constrained settings, and its home–based neonatal care intervention has guided national replication and scale up by the government of India.

CONCLUSIONS

Although there is strong evidence that in highly controlled settings, specific interventions such as hand washing, vitamin A, immunizations and many others can improve child health, there is much less evidence for how health projects in high–mortality, resource–constrained settings can achieve long–lasting impacts on under–five mortality. The common characteristics of the four projects cited here give some important insights in considering this important question.

Most of the evidence regarding the effectiveness of community–based primary health care (CBPHC) in improving maternal, neonatal and chilld health (MNCH) outcomes comes from assessments of the effect of single interventions implemented in highly controlled and atypical field settings over a relatively short period of time, usually five years or less. The four projects identified and described here are the only four in our database of 700 assessments that have evidence of long–term impact of 10 years of more on mortality. The projects described here provide a comprehensive array of child health and maternal and reproductive health services, including family planning. They all provide general curative care, including hospital services, and they all facilitate referral and counter–referral services. Each project uses CHWs and provides strong training and support for them. Each also provides essential services for children in the home, has developed and sustained a high level of community engagement, and has earned the trust of the people it serves.

Each of these projects has used recurrently a cycle of consultation/planning, implementation, reflection/evaluation on a regular basis to adjust their projects to serve the needs of their local population. Over a long time, this process led to project characteristics that have been maintained. The similarity of these four projects' characteristics attests to the strength of this combination of project characteristics in serving its population's health needs.

Building strong and more comprehensive health systems in high–mortality, resource–constrained settings along the lines of the projects described here has the potential for not only long–term improvements in MNHC but also long–term improvements in control of HIV/AIDS, malaria and tuberculosis and even many emerging chronic conditions such as hypertension and diabetes. Learning to build and maintain these systems in a way so that they are affordable with local resources is one of our great challenges.

Acknowledgments: We are grateful to the following people for comments on an earlier version of this paper: Henry Mosely (for comments on the Matlab icddrb section), Gretchen Berggren (for comments on the Hôpital Albert Schweitzer section), Shobha Arole and Connie Gates (for comments on the Jamkhed CRHP section), and Abhay Bang (for comments on the SEARCH/Gadchiroli section). We are grateful to the following organizations that provided small grants to cover the expenses of this review: UNICEF, the World Bank, the Department of Child and Adolescent Health and Development of the World Health Organization, the CORE Group (Collaboration and Resources for Child Health)/USAID, Future Generations, and the Gates Foundation. We are also grateful to the American Public Health Association and particularly its International Health Section staff, which administered some of these funds. We thank Future Generations for providing office space, administrative support, and salary support to Dr Perry during the initial phase of the review. The World Bank made it possible for one of its consultants, Dr Bahie Rassekh, to participate as a member of the Study Team.

Funding: The following organizations provided funds that were used to conduct the work described in this article: The World Health Organization, UNICEF, the World Bank, the United States Agency for International Development, and the Gates Foundation. The organizations that provided financial support had no role in the execution of the review.

Authorship declaration: HP wrote the first draft. All authors reviewed and edited subsequent drafts and approved the final version.

Competing interests: All authors have completed the Unified Competing Interest Form at www.icmje.org/coi_disclosure.pdf (available upon request from the corresponding author), and declare no conflict of interest.

References

1   Perry HB, Rassekh B, Gupta S, Wilhelm J, Freeman P. A comprehensive review of the evidence regarding the effectiveness of community-based primary health care in improving maternal, neonatal and child health: 1. rationale, methods and database description. J Glob Health. 2017;7:010901.

2   Bang AT, Bang RA, Reddy HM. Home-based neonatal care: summary and applications of the field trial in rural Gadchiroli, India (1993 to 2003). J Perinatol. 2005;25 Suppl 1:S108-22. Medline:15791272 doi:10.1038/sj.jp.7211278

3   Perry HB, Cayemittes M, Philippe F, Dowell D, Dortonne JR, Menager H, et al. Reducing under-five mortality through Hopital Albert Schweitzer's integrated system in Haiti. Health Policy Plan. 2006;21:217-30. Medline:16565151 doi:10.1093/heapol/czl005

4   Perry H, Berggren W, Berggren G, Dowell D, Menager H, Bottex E, et al. Long-term reductions in mortality among children under age 5 in rural Haiti: effects of a comprehensive health system in an impoverished setting. Am J Public Health. 2007;97:240-6. Medline:17194853 doi:10.2105/AJPH.2006.088732

5 Arole M, Arole R. Jamkhed – A Comprehensive Rural Health Project. London: Macmillan Press; 1994.

6   Chen LC, Rahman M, D'Souza S, Chakraborty J, Sardar AM, Yunus M. Mortality impact of an MCH-FP program in Matlab, Bangladesh. Stud Fam Plann. 1983;14:199-209. Medline:6636221 doi:10.2307/1966412

7   Razzaque A, Streatfield PK, Gwatkin DR. Does health intervention improve socioeconomic inequalities of neonatal, infant and child mortality? Evidence from Matlab, Bangladesh. Int J Equity Health. 2007;6:4. Medline:17547776 doi:10.1186/1475-9276-6-4

8   Hale L, DaVanzo J, Razzaque A, Rahman M. Why are infant and child mortality rates lower in the MCH-FP area of Matlab, Bangladesh? Stud Fam Plann. 2006;37:281-92. Medline:17209285 doi:10.1111/j.1728-4465.2006.00106.x

9   Aziz K. Mosley H. The History, Methodology, and Main Findings,of the Matlab Project in Bangladesh. In: Das Gupta M, Aaby P, Garenne M, Pison G, editors. Prospective community studies in developing countries International studies in demography. Oxford: Oxford University Press; 1997.

10   Fauveau V. Matlab: Women, Children and Health. Dhaka: International Centre for Diarrhoeal Disease Research, Bangladesh; 1994.

11   icddrb. Matlab and its impact on public health. 2016. Available: http://www.icddrb.org/research/platforms/field-sites/more-on-matlab. Accessed: 26 February 2017.

12   Perry HB. Health for All in Bangladesh: Lessons in Primary Health Care for the Twenty-First Century. Dhaka, Bangladesh: University Press Ltd; 2000.

13   Ali M, Emch M, Tofail F, Baqui AH. Implications of health care provision on acute lower respiratory infection mortality in Bangladeshi children. Soc Sci Med. 2001;52:267-77. Medline:11144783 doi:10.1016/S0277-9536(00)00120-9

14   Mostafa G, Ajmed K, Shaikh MAK, van Ginneken JH, Sarder AM. Demographic Surveillance System – Matlab. Volume 27. Registration of Vital Events – 1995. Dhaka: ICDDR.B.; 1996.

15   Mostafa G, Rahman MM. Demographic Surveillance System – Matlab. Volume 39. Registration of Health and Demographic Events – 2005. Dhaka: ICDDR.B.; 2007.

16   Rahman M, DaVanzo J, Razzaque A. The role of pregnancy outcomes in the maternal mortality rates of two areas in Matlab, Bangladesh. Int Perspect Sex Reprod Health. 2010;36:170-7. Medline:21245023 doi:10.1363/3617010

17 Fauveau V, Chakraborty J. Family Planning and Maternal and Child Health Services in Matlab. Fauveau V, editor. Dhaka: International Centre for Diarrheoal Disease Research, Bangladesh; 1994.

18 World Health Organization. UNICEF. Countdown to 2015 Decade Report (2000-2010) with Country Profiles: Taking Stock of Maternal, Newborn and Child Survival. Geneva: World Health Organization and UNICEF; 2010.

19 El Arifeen S, Christou A, Reichenbach L, Osman FA, Azad K, Islam KS, et al. Community-based approaches and partnerships: innovations in health-service delivery in Bangladesh. Lancet. 2013;382:2012-26. Medline:24268607 doi:10.1016/S0140-6736(13)62149-2

20 Schweitzer HA. Hôpital Albert Schweitzer. 2016. Available: http://www.hashaiti.org/. Accessed: 27 February 2017.

21 Berggren WL, Ewbank DC, Berggren GG. Reduction of mortality in rural Haiti through a primary-health-care program. N Engl J Med. 1981;304:1324-30. Medline:7219486 doi:10.1056/NEJM198105283042203

22 Berggren WL, Berggren GM. Changing incidence of fatal tetanus of the newborn. A retrospective study in a defined rural Haitian populations. Am J Trop Med Hyg. 1971;20:491-4. Medline:5088398 doi:10.4269/ajtmh.1971.20.491

23 Berggren WL. Control of neonatal tetanus in rural Haiti through the utilization of medical auxiliaries. Bull Pan Am Health Organ. 1974;8:24-9. Medline:4423926

24 Perry HB, Northrup R, Bryant J, Berggren W, Berggren G. The cost-effectiveness of a long-term comprehensive primary health care program in reducing under-5 mortality: findings from rural Haiti. J Epidemiol Community Health. Forthcoming 2017.

25 Victora CG, Requejo JH, Barros AJ, Berman P, Bhutta Z, Boerma T, et al. Countdown to 2015: a decade of tracking progress for maternal, newborn, and child survival. Lancet. 2016;387:2049-59. Medline:26477328 doi:10.1016/S0140-6736(15)00519-X

26 Jamkhed Comprehensive Rural Health Project. Comprehensive Rural Health Project Impact. 2016. Available: http://www.crhpjamkhed.org/impact/impact. Accessed: 27 February 2017.

27 Ministry of Health and Family Welfare GoI. Maharashtra: National Family Health Survey (NFHS-3), India, 2005-06. Mumbai, India: International Institute for Population Sciences; 2007. Available: http://www.nfhsindia.org/NFHS-3%20Data/Maharashtra_report.pdf. Accessed: 26 February 2017.

28 Mann V, Eble A, Frost C, Premkumar R, Boone P. Retrospective comparative evaluation of the lasting impact of a community-based primary health care programme on under-5 mortality in villages around Jamkhed, India. Bull World Health Organ. 2010;88:727-36. Medline:20931057 doi:10.2471/BLT.09.064469

29 McCord C, Premkumar R, Arole S, Arole R. Efficient and effective emergency obstetric care in a rural Indian community where most deliveries are at home. Int J Gynaecol Obstet. 2001;75:297-307, discussion 8-9. Medline:11728493 doi:10.1016/S0020-7292(01)00526-4

30 Newell KW, editor. Health by the People. Geneva: World Health Organization; 1975.

31 Arole M, Arole R. A comprehensive rural health project in Jamkhed (India). In: Newell KW, editor. Health by the People. Geneva, Switzerland: World Health Organization; 1975.

32 SEARCH. Society for Education, Action and Research in Community Health. 2016. Available: http://www.searchgadchiroli.org/. Accessed: 26 February 2017.

33 Dasgupta D. SEARCH: Society for Education, Action and Research in Community Health. Delhi: Voluntary Health Association of India; 1998.

34 Bang AT, Bang RA. Background of the field trial of home-based neonatal care in Gadchiroli, India. J Perinatol. 2005;25 Suppl 1:S3-10. Medline:15791276 doi:10.1038/sj.jp.7211267

35 Kielmann AA, Taylor CE, DeSweemer C, Parker RL. D. C, Reinke WA, et al. Volume 1. Child and Maternal Health Services in Rural India: the Narangwal Experiment. Integrated Nutrition and Health Care. Baltimore: Published for the World Bank [by] Johns Hopkins University Press; 1983.

36 Taylor CE, Sarma RSS, Parker RL, Reinke WA, Faruqee R. Volume 2. Child and Maternal Health Services in Rural India: the Narangwal Experiment. Integrated Family Planning and Health Care. Baltimore, MD: Johns Hopkins University Press; 1983.

37 Bang A, Bang R. Addiction as a barrier to development. In: Taylor-Ide D, Taylor C, editors. Just and Lasting Change: When Communities Own Their Futures. Baltimore: Johns Hopkins University Press; 2002.

38 Bang AT, Bang RA, Tale O, Sontakke P, Solanki J, Wargantiwar R, et al. Reduction in pneumonia mortality and total childhood mortality by means of community-based intervention trial in Gadchiroli, India. Lancet. 1990;336:201-6. Medline:1973770 doi:10.1016/0140-6736(90)91733-Q

39 Bang AT, Reddy HM, Deshmukh MD, Baitule SB, Bang RA. Neonatal and infant mortality in the ten years (1993 to 2003) of the Gadchiroli field trial: effect of home-based neonatal care. J Perinatol. 2005;25 Suppl 1:S92-107. Medline:15791283 doi:10.1038/sj.jp.7211277

40 Bang AT, Bang RA, Baitule SB, Reddy MH, Deshmukh MD. Effect of home-based neonatal care and management of sepsis on neonatal mortality: field trial in rural India. Lancet. 1999;354:1955-61. Medline:10622298 doi:10.1016/S0140-6736(99)03046-9

41 Perry H, Scott K, Javadi D, Gergen J, Shelley K, Crigler L, et al. Case Studies of Large-Scale Community Health Worker Programs: Examples from Afghanistan, Bangladesh, Brazil, Ethiopia, India, Indonesia, Iran, Nepal, Niger, Pakistan, Rwanda, Zambia, and Zimbabwe. 2017. Washington, DC: USAID/MCSP. Available: http://www.mcsprogram.org/wp-content/uploads/2017/01/CHW-CaseStudies-Globes.pdf. Accessed: 26 February 2017.

42 Wyon JB, Gordon JE. The Khanna Study: Population Problems in the Rural Punjab. Cambridge, MA: Harvard University Press; 1971.

Acknowledgement: originally published as: Henry B Perry, Bahie M Rassekh, Sundeep Gupta, Paul A Freeman:Comprehensive review of the evidence regarding the effectiveness of Community–Based Primary Health Care in improving maternal, neonatal and child health: 7. strategies used by effective projects. Reprinted with permission from Edinburgh University Global Health Society under Creative Commons Attribution Licence (Journal of Global Health 2017; 010907).

Comprehensive review of the evidence regarding the effectiveness of community–based primary health care in improving maternal, neonatal and child health: 8. summary and recommendations of the Expert Panel

Robert E Black[1,*], Carl E Taylor[1,†], Shobha Arole[2,*,‡], Abhay Bang[3,*,‡], Zulfiqar A Bhutta[4,5,*,‡], A Mushtaque R Chowdhury[6,*,‡], Betty R Kirkwood[7,*,‡], Nazo Kureshy[8,*,‡], Claudio F Lanata[9,*,‡], James F Phillips[10,*,‡], Mary Taylor[11,*,‡], Cesar G Victora[12,*,‡], Zonghan Zhu[13,*,‡], Henry B Perry[1]

---

[1] Johns Hopkins Bloomberg School of Public Health, Baltimore, Maryland, USA
[2] Jamkhed Comprehensive Rural Health Project, Jamkhed, Maharashtra, India
[3] Society for Education, Action and Research in Community Health, Gadchiroli, Maharashtra, India
[4] University of Toronto, Toronto, Ontario, Canada
[5] Aga Khan University, Karachi, Pakistan
[6] BRAC, Dhaka, Bangladesh
[7] London School of Hygiene and Tropical Medicine, London, United Kingdom
[8] Bureau of Global Health, United States Agency for International Development, Washington, DC, USA
[9] Institute of Nutritional Research, Lima, Peru
[10] Columbia University Mailman School of Public Health, New York, New York, USA
[11] Independent Consultant, South Royalton, Vermont, USA
[12] Federal University of Pelotas, Pelotas, Brazil
[13] Capital Institute of Pediatrics and China Advisory Center for Child Health, Beijing, China
[*] Chairperson, Expert Panel
[†] Former Chairperson, Expert Panel (deceased)
[‡] Member, Expert Panel

Background The contributions that community–based primary health care (CB-PHC) and engaging with communities as valued partners can make to the improvement of maternal, neonatal and child health (MNCH) is not widely appreciated. This unfortunate reality is one of the reasons why so few priority countries failed to achieve the health–related Millennium Development Goals by 2015. This article provides a summary of a series of articles about the effectiveness of CBPHC in improving MNCH and offers recommendations from an Expert Panel for strengthening CBPHC that were formulated in 2008 and have been updated on the basis of more recent evidence.

Methods An Expert Panel convened to guide the review of the effectiveness of community–based primary health care (CBPHC). The Expert Panel met in 2008 in New York City with senior UNICEF staff. In 2016, following the completion of the review, the Panel considered the review's findings and made recommendations. The review consisted of an analysis of 661 unique reports, including 583 peer–reviewed journal articles, 12 books/monographs, 4 book chapters, and 72 reports from the gray literature. The analysis consisted of 700 assessments since 39 were analyzed twice (once for an assessment of improvements in neonatal and/ or child health and once for an assessment in maternal health).

Results The Expert Panel recommends that CBPHC should be a priority for strengthening health systems, accelerating progress in achieving universal health coverage, and ending preventable child and maternal deaths. The Panel also recommends that expenditures for CBPHC be monitored against expenditures for primary health care facilities and hospitals and reflect the importance of CBPHC for averting mortality. Governments, government health programs, and NGOs should develop health systems that respect and value communities as full partners and work collaboratively with them in building and strengthening CBPHC programs – through engagement with planning, implementation (including the full use of community–level workers), and evaluation. CBPHC programs need to reach every community and household in order to achieve universal coverage of key evidence–based interventions that can be implemented in the community outside of health facilities and assure that those most in need are reached.

Conclusions Stronger CBPHC programs that foster community engagement/ empowerment with the implementation of evidence–based interventions will be essential for achieving universal coverage of health services by 2030 (as called for by the Sustainable Development Goals recently adopted by the United Nations), ending preventable child and maternal deaths by 2030 (as called for by the World Health Organization, UNICEF, and many countries around the world), and eventually achieving Health for All as envisioned at the International Conference on Primary Health Care in 1978. Stronger CBPHC programs can also create entry points and synergies for expanding the coverage of family planning services as well as for accelerating progress in the detection and treatment of HIV/AIDS, tuberculosis, malaria, hypertension, and other chronic diseases. Continued strengthening of CBPHC programs based on rigorous ongoing operations research and evaluation will be required, and this evidence will be needed to guide national and international policies and programs.

This paper summarizes the current evidence regarding the effectiveness of community–based primary health care (CBPHC) in improving maternal, neonatal and child health (MNCH). It also proposes concrete steps to recognize that communities are a vital resource and key partners with health systems in improving MNCH.

We summarize here the findings presented in the earlier articles in this current series [1–7] and in the Reproductive, Maternal, Newborn and Child Health volume of the Disease Control Priorities, Third Edition [8,9]. It also is an outgrowth of the Working Group on CBPHC of the International Health Section of the American Public Health Association, and the papers of the Working Group prepared previously [10–12] as well as discussions of an Expert Panel (for membership see **Online Supplementary Document**) convened to guide the activities of the Working Group when the Panel met at UNICEF headquarters in New York City on 27–8 March 2008 with senior UNICEF staff along with senior staff from the World Health Organization (WHO) and the World Bank.

CBPHC is defined as a process by which health systems work with communities to improve health through activities that may be linked with health facilities but which take place in communities. The role of communities and community–based approaches to improving MNCH is still being overshadowed by the traditional "facility–centric" approach to health systems and calls for a new paradigm in which communities and community–based services are brought to the mainstream of health programs in order to improve the effectiveness of health systems in resource–constrained settings. Hybrid approaches also need to be developed in which professionalized CHWs divide their time by attending to patients at a village–based health post and visiting families in their homes, as is the case in Ethiopia.

The previous articles in this series provide an in–depth comprehensive review of evidence accumulated for over half a century regarding the effectiveness of community–based primary health care (CBPHC) in improving maternal, neonatal and child health (MNCH). The authors identified assessments of the health effects of community–based projects, programs and research studies (hereafter referred to as projects) in defined geographic populations. The review defines health effects broadly: change in (1) the population coverage of evidence–based interventions, (2) nutritional status, (3) serious morbidity, and (4) mortality. Not only did the authors assess health effects, but they also examined the equity of these projects as well as the strategies used to achieve health effects, including the common strategies of four projects identified that had evidence of mortality impact for 10 years or longer.

Why the review is important now

The era of the Millennium Development Goals (MDGs) ended in 2015 with only seven of 75 Countdown countries reaching the goal for maternal mortality and only one–third reaching the goal for mortality of children younger than five years of age [8]. The population coverage of 13 of 21 key evidence–based MNCH interventions is still less than 60% and for 6 of the 21 interventions it is less than 40% [8]. The second international *Countdown to 2015 Conference* met in Cape Town, South Africa, on 17–19 April 2008. The Call for Action arising from this Conference focused on the need for "long–term, predictable financing for strengthened health systems to deliver essential services to women, newborns and children," "dramatic scale–up of high–impact interventions," harmonization of donor support, and increased political commitment to health around the world [9]. However, there was no mention or call for building stronger partnerships with communities or strengthening CBPHC. Communities are the most undervalued resource in global health. Had communities been engaged more fully as partners with health systems, and had community–based primary health care been more fully developed, we believe there is a strong possibility that the MDG era might have ended very differently.

In 1948, the United Nations General Assembly affirmed in its Universal Declaration of Human Rights that everyone has a right to medical care and that "motherhood and childhood are entitled to special care and assistance" [13]. Forty years later, in 1978, the largest gathering of health officials convened up to that time by the World Health Organization and UNICEF affirmed at the International Conference on Primary Health Care that an acceptable level of health for all the people of the world could be achieved by the year 2000 through a fuller and better use of the world's resources (see **Box 1**) [15]. As the world seeks still to achieve these lofty goals, much work remains to be done. In 2015 the United Nations has adopted the Sustainable Development Goals, calling for a world *"free of poverty, hunger, disease and want, where all lives can thrive"* by the year 2030, with universal access to *"quality essential health–care services"* [16]. The World Health Organization and UNICEF have called for ending preventable child and maternal deaths in a generation [17,18]. However, even though recently released plans for achieving this goal do emphasize

Box 1. *The Declaration of Alma Ata*

"The people have the right and duty to participate individually and collectively in the planning and implementation of their health care" (Article V).

"Primary health care is essential health care based on practical, scientifically sound and socially acceptable methods and technology made universally accessible to individuals and families in the community through their full participation and at a cost that the community and country can afford to maintain at every stage of their development in the spirit of self–reliance and self–determination" (Article VI).

Primary health care "requires and promotes maximum community and individual self–reliance and participation in the planning, organization, operation and control of primary health care, making fullest use of local, national and other available resources; and to this end develops through appropriate education the ability of communities to participate" (Article VII) [14].

the importance of community engagement/empowerment, the critical and fundamental contribution of CBPHC to achieving this goal is muted [19,20].

RESULTS

Specific interventions

Table 1 contains the evidence–based interventions that can be provided by community–level workers with appropriate training, supervision and support.

Table 1. *Effective interventions for maternal, newborn and child health that can be provided by community health workers in the community or at a health post [21–23]*

POINT IN CONTINUUM OF CARE				
Pregnancy	**Delivery (normal)**	**Postpartum (woman)**	**Postpartum (newborn)**	**Child**
Preparation for safe birth and newborn care; emergency planning	Management of labor and delivery and referral of complications	Promotion of breastfeeding	Neonatal resuscitation	Promote breastfeeding and complementary feeding
Micronutrient supplementation*			Breastfeeding	Provide vitamin A, zinc, and food supplementation
Nutrition education			Thermal care for preterm newborns	Immunizations
Intermittent preventive treatment of malaria during pregnancy)			Promote care–seeking	Co–trimoxazole for HIV–positive children
Food supplementation			Assess for danger signs and refer	Education on safe disposal of children's stools and handwashing
Promotion of HIV testing			Oral antibiotics for pneumonia	Distribute and promote use of ITNs† or IRS‡, or both
				Assess for danger signs and refer
				Detect and refer children with severe acute malnutrition
				Detect and treat serious infections without danger signs (iCCM§), refer if danger signs present

*Because of some evidence of risk and gaps in the evidence, the WHO does not at this time recommend multiple micronutrient supplementation for pregnant women to improve maternal and perinatal outcomes [24].

†Insecticide–treated bednet.

‡Indoor residual spraying.

§Integrated community case management (the components include treatments for diarrhea, pneumonia, malaria).

All of these interventions are described in the review. The number of such interventions will certainly continue to grow with continued experience and operations research.

Equity

Although the equity of CBPHC services have not been studied as extensively as has overall intervention effectiveness, the available evidence supports a strong pro–equity effect of CBPHC interventions, as described in more detail in Paper 5 of this series [5]. The term pro–equity effect signifies that the most disadvantaged segment of the population, usually defined in terms of income quintiles or some other type of socio–economic status, benefit more from the delivery of one or more CBPHC interventions than does the better–off segment of the population. Community–based approaches can reach those furthest from health facilities and can rapidly expand population coverage of key interventions, so these findings are not surprising. These findings stand in stark contrast to the commonly observed finding that utilization of primary health care facilities is inequitable because those in the lower income quintiles are less likely to obtain services there [25,26]. This evidence together with the lack of evidence that investments in facilities alone can improve population health in resource–constrained settings [27,28] provide additional support for the importance of investing in CBPHC for improving MNCH.

Strategies for achieving effectiveness

The projects included in the review utilized myriad innovative approaches for working in partnership with communities and with health systems for making CBPHC interventions effective in improving MNCH. These are described in greater detail in paper 4 in this series [6]. Clearly no one size fits all situations, and contextual considerations have a major influence on project operations. Nevertheless, important themes emerged from the review. Many project assessments described engagement with community leaders (both formal and informal), engagement with existing and/or formation of new women's groups, and devising innovative ways to share key education messages with the community (through skits, songs, stories, games and peer–to–peer education). Community–level workers of many types (including both volunteer and paid workers) assisted with project implementation. In most cases, these workers were women, and in three–quarters of the projects included in the review some type of training was provided to these workers. In more than half the projects assessed the community was involved in project implementation, promotion of partnerships between the project and the community, promotion of the use of local resources, and promotion of community engagement/empowerment. In nearly half of the projects, promotion of women's empowerment was present. In approximately 39% of the projects, communities were involved in planning the project and in 40% they were involved in the evaluation.

Many projects engaged in health system strengthening activities of various types, including training of staff based at peripheral health facilities who supervise community–level activities and treat referred patients, strengthening the supervisory system of community–level workers and the logistics/drug supply system for both the peripheral health facility and the community–level workers, and strengthening the referral system. Building strong links among the community–level activities, the peripheral health facility and the referral hospital were common features of effective projects.

Finally, four implementation intervention strategies were commonly encountered. First, home visitations, often routine visits to all homes as well as visits to targeted groups, were often carried out by both volunteer and paid community–level workers. Second, these workers commonly provided community case management, in which they provided education on warning and dangers signs, identified cases in need of referral, and/or treated cases in the community with appropriate medications. A third strategy identified among the projects included in the assessments was the formation of participatory women's groups in which groups of women meet with a facilitator to learn about ways in which they can promote their own health and the health of their children and share this information in their community. The process not only improves the health of mothers and children but it empowers women at the same time. A fourth implementation strategy identified is the provision of community–based services by mobile teams based a peripheral health facilities. These four strategies are not mutually exclusive, of course.

Of the 700 assessments, only four had evidence of mortality impact of 10 years or more, but their common features are striking: they all provided a comprehensive set of primary health care services, including family planning; they had a strong community health worker program that maintained regular contact with all households; they all had strong collaborations with the communities they serve; and they all had strong referral capabilities and provided first–level hospital care.

Limitations of the evidence identified

Although the evidence is extensive, it does have important limitations that need to be recognized. First of all, the evidence is largely limited to assessments of a small number of interventions implemented over a relatively short period of time (2–3 years) in highly controlled field settings with a relatively small population (only 11% of the projects assessed served more than 25 000 women and children), and almost half (46%) of the projects were implemented over a period of 1 year or less and with only 13% implemented over a period of 5 or more years. Thus, the evidence for effectiveness of more comprehensive programs that reach larger populations over longer periods of time is limited.

There is a notable lack of evidence regarding failed attempts to improve MNCH through CBPHC. Publication bias needs to be recognized, and the overall findings interpreted accordingly. But more importantly, more analyses are needed of the main barriers that hinder the fuller development of CBPHC to improve MNCH and steps that need to be taken to overcome them. Furthermore, more attention needs to be given to the puzzling question of why, given the overwhelming evidence, more effort has not been given to strengthening and scaling up CBPHC, especially in countries with a high burden of maternal, neonatal and child mortality. Ghana is a case in point, where an effective evidence–based CBPHC approach [29] reached only 8% national coverage over an 8–year period as a result of inadequate financial backing and donor support [30,31].

We make no claim that this is a systematic review of the evidence. We do claim that it is a comprehensive review of the evidence. The presence of an *a priori* design, the inclusion of gray literature, the listing of included articles, the presence of a quality assessment of included reviews and incorporation of this into conclusions of individual articles, and the inclusion of conflict of interest and funding information for the entire review allow the review to meet 7 of the 11 quality AMSTAR criteria for judging the quality of a systematic review [32].

Given the broad scope and heterogeneity of the evidence included, by necessity the review is largely descriptive and does not undertake a quantitative analysis of effect strength of specific interventions or packages of interventions. This limits the power of conclusions that pertain to specific interventions. Nonetheless, the main finding of the review, namely that CBPHC is an effective and essential approach for improving MNCH, is not lost by dwelling on detailed discussions of which specific interventions or which packages of interventions are most important. We know that new interventions will continually be introduced in the future, and epidemiological as well contextual conditions will change over time, so keeping a focus on CBPHC as a strategy for implementing specific interventions, which this review attempts to do, is important.

Strengths of the review

The review described in this series has some important strengths. First, it is one of the most comprehensive in–depth current reviews on this important topic that is highly relevant for accelerating progress in reducing 6 million deaths of mothers and their offspring each year [8,9], most of which are from readily preventable or treatable conditions. While the effectiveness of many of the interventions described here is well–known, the breadth of interventions known to be effective is less well–known, as are the most common strategies used to implement them. The reviewers included evidence not only from the peer–reviewed literature but also from unpublished project evaluations, books, and reports from the gray literature. The review is composed of 700 assessments. Second, it is one of the most comprehensive reviews currently available, with great efforts taken to extract all available information about how each project included in the review was implemented, how communities were engaged, how interventions were delivered at the community level, and what steps were taken to strengthen the health system.

Estimates of the number of lives of mothers and their children that could be saved by scaling up CBPHC

Long–standing experience and rapidly growing evidence both show that simplified home– and community–based interventions can be remarkably effective in expanding the coverage of evidence–based interventions and reducing maternal, neonatal and child mortality [22,23]. The best current evidence indicates that if the complete package of evidence–based interventions for mothers and their children that can be provided at the community level reach all who need them, 2.3 million deaths would be averted each year compared to the interventions that require delivery in primary health care centers (which would avert 0.8 million deaths) and in hospitals (which would avert 0.9 million deaths) (**Figure 1**) [22].

Promoting community engagement/empowerment

Promoting community engagement/empowerment to increase intervention effectiveness is obviously not simple, but major progress has been documented [33]. Experience shows that the following questions must be addressed by both programs and communities:
   • Will the community be a participating partner and bring its own considerable resources (mostly non–financial) to improve MNCH, or will the more

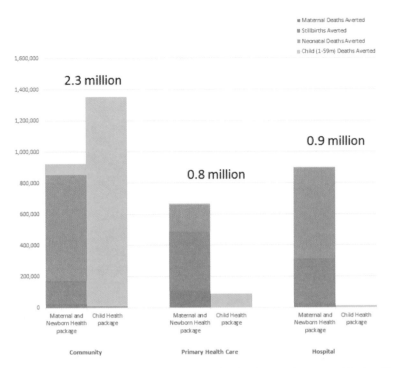

Figure 1. Maternal, perinatal, neonatal and child deaths that can be averted by health–care packages through three service platforms [22]. The numbers above the columns were not in the original figure. The services assumed to be provided in each platform are as follows. *The community platform:* all interventions that can be delivered by a community–based health worker with appropriate training and support or by outreach services, such as child health days, immunizations, vitamin A, and other interventions. *The primary health center (PHC) platform:* a facility with a doctor or a nurse midwife (or both), nurses and support staff, as well as both diagnostic and treatment capabilities. The PHC provides facility–based contraceptive services, including long–acting reversible contraceptives (implants, intra-uterine devices); surgical sterilization (vasectomy, tubal ligation); care during pregnancy and delivery for uncomplicated pregnancies; provision of medical care for adults and children, such as injectable antibiotics, that cannot be done in the community; and training and supervision of community–based workers. *The hospital platform:* consisting of both first–level and referral hospitals, includes more advanced services for management of labor and delivery in high–risk women or those with complications, including operative delivery, full supportive care for preterm newborns, and care of children with severe infection or severe acute malnutrition with infection [22].

common practices continue of health systems considering communities mainly as targets and essentially passive recipients of services?

- Will the community have the opportunity to participate in setting priorities as well as implementing and evaluating program activities, in contrast to the much more common practice of health professionals defining these roles as the responsibility of the health system?

Although the Expert Panel did not approach these questions as either–or alternatives, it did view community engagement/empowerment as important for enabling the delivery system to more effectively improve MNCH.

Activities that communities can contribute to improving the effectiveness of interventions and that can be empowering for communities include the following:

- Involving local leadership in mobilizing the community for planning and management of activities (including the management of external resources);
- Clarifying local value systems to help both the delivery system and community develop mutual understanding and respect as they work together for results that are effective and equitable;
- Involving women's groups in participatory learning and action, peer–to–peer education, and provision of home–based care;
- Involving men and mothers–in–law in creative ways that encourage healthy behaviors and appropriate health care utilization;
- Participating in adapting the delivery system to local realities and local culture with integration of interventions for acceptability and efficiency;
- Participating in monitoring, evaluation and accountability; and,
- Collaborating not just in a series of interventions during the initial stages of implementation but establishing long–term partnerships for robust and sustainable systems.

Effective program planning, implementation and assessment require community involvement, and the evidence is clearest for home–based neonatal care and community–based management of childhood diarrhea, pneumonia and malaria. For other interventions (eg, immunizations), community engagement/empowerment is important to ensure that children who need an intervention are taken to where they can receive it (or to take the intervention to where the child is, ie, in the home). CBPHC requires linkages with facilities. Populations with the most limited access to formal health care are typically in the most unreached areas where mortality is the highest and therefore where impact can be greatest. Here also equity issues are central. The nature of effective partnerships between health intervention delivery systems and communities vary greatly as a result of the need to adapt them to the local context [34]. Supportive environments for CBPHC and community engagement/empowerment at local, national, international and global levels are now needed, especially as the evidence of effectiveness continues to grow. Community–level workers providing CBPHC have been shown to be effective in improving not only MNCH in low–income countries but also in improving health priorities in middle– and upper–income countries as well [35,36].

Scaling up community–based primary health care

The evidence for the effectiveness of CBPHC in improving MNCH at scale is still limited. Yet, encouraging national examples of improvement in MNCH exist in countries such as Afghanistan, Brazil, Ethiopia, Nepal and Rwanda [37,38] and these countries have established strong CBPHC programs that have made a major contribution to these achievements. More research is needed to fully assess the contribution that strengthened CBPHC has made to these achievements.

Innovative approaches to scaling up CBPHC approaches that improve MNCH are needed. Some examples are the following:

- Establishment of a cadre of government–authorized community–level workers throughout the country with gradual addition of responsibilities, as has happened in Afghanistan, Brazil, Bangladesh, Ethiopia, India, Malawi, Nepal, Niger, Rwanda, and many other countries [38];
- The gradual expansion of a package of interventions to national level beginning with a small effective program implemented by one NGO, replication by other NGOs, with gradual transfer of the intervention into the government system as is currently underway in India, as has occurred for home–based neonatal care, beginning with SEARCH's pioneering work in Gadchiroli [39];
- "Scaling down to scale up" in which a documented successful approach is replicated at other sites with strong local input and flexibility, allowing local champions to emerge, as has been carried out by the Navrongo Initiative working through the Ministry of Health in Ghana [29];
- A three–way partnership at the outset for scaling up, in which the community, government officials, and an outside agent (such as an NGO or technical support group) first establishes model program sites as nodes to adapt and systematize extension to larger populations, as was done in China with the Model Counties Project [40] (which has now become China's rural MCH system) and as Future Generations has done with its SEED–SCALE approach to improve the health of children in Arunachal Pradesh (India); Tibet (China), Afghanistan and Peru [41];
- A "bottom–up" educational approach to scaling up, in which grassroots workers from many geographic areas and programs in different countries come to a central training center to learn empowerment and CBPHC, as is occurring at the Comprehensive Rural Health Program (CRHP) in Jamkhed, India, where more than 30 000 people from around India and more than 3000 people from 100 other countries have now been trained [42];

- Creation of a national framework giving local communities the option of establishing shared control over health centers and local programs, as has occurred in Peru's program of *Communidades Locales para la Administracion de Salud* (CLAS), under which one–third of the government's 2400 health centers are now governed [43]; and,

- The gradual expansion of one key intervention to a national level under the direction of a single NGO, as was carried out by BRAC through its home–based training of mothers to prevent and treat childhood diarrhea [44].

There is a need to test different approaches for rapid scaling up so that CBPHC programs can achieve national impact more rapidly. Even though "command and control" approaches can be used for scaling up standardized components of community–based interventions, in most poor countries such approaches have been supported by external donors for only a limited time period, producing initial successes that cannot be sustained after external funding ends. By contrast, new systematic processes need to be developed that can adapt to local realities in ways that promote community engagement/empowerment and long–term local sustainability [25]. Different approaches to scaling up should be tested through monitoring of quality and coverage as well as through rigorous implementation research. This would enhance the potential for greater effectiveness and long–term sustainability without over–dependence on central or international funding.

The limited evidence of effectiveness of a broad package of CBPHC interventions over a period of more than 3 years at scale is a serious concern. Long–term field studies to assess the ongoing effectiveness of a comprehensive package of CBPHC interventions are needed to enable such programs to continually improve their effectiveness and to provide guidance for similar programs. The strengthening and scaling up of effective CBPHC programs is a long–term process that will require continuing adjustment as conditions and contexts change, and as new evidence-based interventions become available. Efficiencies and final aspects of CBPHC are not adequately address in the literature. Thus, investments in long–term implementation research are greatly needed.

Specific recommendations of the Expert Panel

The Expert Panel calls for the following steps.
1. CBPHC should be a priority for strengthening health systems, for accelerating progress in achieving universal health coverage, and for ending preventable child and maternal deaths.

2. The amount of resources devoted to CBPHC should be tracked at national and regional levels, and attention should be given by policy makers and political leaders to ensure that funding for CBPHC is expanding appropriately.

3. Communities are an undervalued resource, and their full participation and partnership needs to be fostered in order for CBPHC to reach its full potential. Building partnerships between health systems and communities is essential in order to reach those most in need with effective, equitable, and sustainable programs.

4. Prioritization should be given to strengthening CBPHC in populations with the highest mortality in order to achieve greater impact.

5. A strong CBPHC service delivery platform should be established not only for accelerating progress in improving MNCH and child development but also for reducing the unmet need for family planning, for ending the HIV/AIDS epidemic, controlling malaria, tuberculosis, and priority non–communicable diseases such as hypertension, diabetes and mental illness, and for surveillance (identification of infectious disease outbreaks and registration of vital events). The establishment of the CBHC service delivery platform for MNCH is urgent, while the inclusion of other elements will need to be a gradual and longer–term process. A strong CBPHC service delivery system will make it possible to incorporate new interventions as they are developed, and such a system will be needed for the long term, even after ending preventable child and maternal deaths and achieving universal coverage of health services. Such a system will be needed, in fact, for eventually reaching universal comprehensive health coverage and Health for All.

6. Future progress in improving the effectiveness of CBPHC for MNCH will require an expanded research agenda to continually advance the contextualized evidence on CBPHC program effectiveness at scale over a longer period of time with multiple evidence–based interventions. Adequate financial support for advancing the evidence base for CBPHC program effectiveness will be essential if CBPHC programs are to fulfill their potential.

Table 2 and **Table 3** provide additional detailed to the recommendations of the Expert Panel for promoting community engagement/empowerment and for strengthening health systems that will make it possible for CBPHC to more effectively reduce maternal, neonatal and child mortality.

Reaching the unreached and most vulnerable members of our global family – namely mothers and children – through CBPHC was the vision of the three

Table 2. *Expert Panel recommendations for promoting community engagement/empowerment for improved maternal, neonatal and child health*

Main recommendations	Details
Empower communities and women in these communities to be more actively engaged in improving the health of mothers, newborns and children	Establish a foundation of values that supports partnerships with communities and processes to build community capacity through giving communities a voice in supervising or controlling certain aspects of local government health services, and through building the agency of women (such as the promotion of women's empowerment, support of micro–credit programs and development of conditional cash transfer programs).
	Support the development of community–based organizations focused on local health needs and on the planning, implementation, and evaluation of local health programs.
Build stronger partnerships between the community and the health system	Create a health system culture that is respectful of and collaborative with community members.
	Create bi–directional communication flows.
	Create bi–directional linkages between the district health system and communities that can help everyone be accountable for health system performance.
Involve communities in monitoring, evaluation, and use of health–related information	Create systems for the community's generation and use of health data (including registration of births and deaths and identification of those in greatest need of services, as part of a continuing process to promote equity in all stages of health care).
	Develop participatory approaches to the monitoring and evaluation of CBPHC programs, including assessments of mortality impact.

Table 3. *Expert Panel recommendations for strengthening the delivery system for improved maternal, neonatal and child health*

Main recommendations	Details
Extend the delivery system to every community and household	Involve community members in the delivery of services.
	Train and support community–level workers who (1) receive sufficient incentives or salary to support their long–term involvement, (2) receive appropriate supportive and technical supervision from staff based at the nearest health facility, and (3) are accountable to their local community.
	Provide appropriate training and supervision of community–level workers (who preferably are selected from and by the communities where they will work) to perform health tasks that respond to local health needs and that address the epidemiological priorities of mothers and their children.
	Train and support neighborhood volunteers for peer–to–peer health promotion.
	Develop an appropriate balance of community–level workers for the required service intensity (while at the same time ensuring a suitable workload for an appropriate number of tasks and ensuring enough time required for each task, given the distance to homes and the level of remuneration/ incentives).

Table 3. *Continued*

MAIN RECOMMENDATIONS	DETAILS
	Coordinate the activities of the formal health sector with the informal health sector (drug sellers and individual practitioners, including traditional healers).
Promote delivery of interventions to those at greatest risk	Provide "safety nets" that reduce barriers to accessing and providing services (eg, "CBPHC–friendly" insurance systems to remunerate providers and incentive schemes to promote utilization of health services).
	Create equitable service delivery strategies that identify and reach those in greatest need
Build a stronger, more efficient, and more effective health delivery system	Provide adequate, sustainable and flexible global, national and local financing that responds to the needs of community–based programs in relation to the amount being spent for facility–based care.
	Foster investments at the community and local level for support of community–based programs and for strengthening primary health care at peripheral health facilities.
	Provide adequate supplies for service delivery.
	Integrate services at the community level (based on delivery system capacity and local need).
	Monitor expenditures for CBPHC against those for primary health centers and hospitals and ensure that these levels are appropriate given the importance of CBPHC for averting deaths.

global health pioneers – Carl Taylor (founder of the Department of International Health at Johns Hopkins and Chair of the Expert Panel prior to his death in 2010), Jim Grant (Executive Director of UNICEF from 1980 to 1995) and Halfdan Mahler (Director General of WHO from 1973–1988). They all provided leadership for the International Conference on Primary Health Care at Alma–Ata in 1978 and its Declaration of Alma–Ata and worked tirelessly to achieve that vision, which remains unfilled. They recognized, and the Declaration of Alma–Ata affirms, that health care needs to be brought "as close as possible to where people live and work" and that this requires health workers at all levels, including *"physicians, nurses, midwives, auxiliaries and community workers as applicable"* [14]. Over the past three decades, the evidence of what can be achieved through CBPHC to improve the health of mothers, neonates and children has grown exponentially.

However, CBPHC still remains, as El–Saharty and colleagues rightly calls it, an "unfunded afterthought" [45] (p. 270) rather than the solid foundation of effective health systems. Jim Grant repeatedly reminded us that "morality must march with changing capacity" [46]. And Halfdan Mahler reminded the world in his 2008 address to the 61st World Health Assembly, "unless we all become partisans in the renewed local and global battles for social and economic equity in the spirit of distributive justice, we shall indeed betray the future of our children and grandchildren" [47]. Establishing the political will to fund and build strong CBPHC programs is urgently needed, as is defining the resource needs so that these programs will not remain an "unfunded afterthought."

Carl Taylor, in his final publication, wrote that "[r]eal social change occurs when officials and people with relevant knowledge and resources come together with communities in joint action around mutual priorities" [34]. The evidence confirms the promise of CBPHC in ending preventable maternal, neonatal and child deaths. Building on this evidence and making CBPHC the priority that it needs to be is one of the great challenges for global health in the 21st century and one of the giant steps that can be taken to eventually achieve Health for All.

CONCLUSIONS

Stronger CBPHC programs that foster community engagement/empowerment and implement evidence–based interventions will be essential for achieving universal coverage of health services by 2030 (as called for by the Sustainable Development Goals recently adopted by the United Nations) [48]), ending preventable child and maternal deaths by 2030 (as called for by the World Health Organization, UNICEF and many other countries) [17], and eventually achieving Health for All as initially envisioned in 1978 at the International Conference on Primary Health Care convened by WHO and UNICEF [14]. Stronger CBPHC programs will create entry points and synergies for expanding the coverage of family planning services [49] and for accelerating progress in the detection and treatment of HIV/AIDS [50], tuberculosis [51] malaria [52], and hypertension and other chronic diseases [53]. International cooperation will be important in promoting stronger CBPHC implementation world–wide. Advocacy at global, international, national and local levels, exchange of information and experiences, training, and evaluations of program implementation will all contribute to stronger CBPHC programming. Specific mechanisms need to be developed through which we can more effectively learn from experience and generate evidence to guide local, national and international policies and programs.

Acknowledgments: *The authors express the gratitude and indebtedness to the late Dr Carl E. Taylor for his lifetime of leadership in community–based primary health care, his early support of this project, and his leadership as Chair of the Expert Panel until his death in 2010.*

Funding: *None.*

Authorship *declaration: HP and RB wrote the first draft. All of the authors participated in a revision of first draft and approved the final draft.*

Conflict *of interest*: *All authors have completed the Unified Competing Interest Form at www.icmje.org/coi_disclosure.pdf (available upon request from the corresponding author), and declare no conflict of interest. Nazo Kureshy's participation as a member of the Expert Panel was as an individual, not as an official representative of the United States Agency for International Development (USAID), and the views expressed in this paper are not official views of USAID.*

References

1 Perry H, Rassekh B, Gupta S, Wilhelm J, Freeman P. Comprehensive review of the evidence regarding the effectiveness of community-based primary health care in improving maternal, neonatal and child health: 1. rationale, methods and database description. J Glob Health. 2017;7:010901.

2 Jennings M, Pradhan S, Schleiff M, Sacks E, Freeman P, Gupta S, et al. Comprehensive review of the evidence regarding the effectiveness of community-based primary health care in improving maternal, neonatal and child health: 2. maternal health findings. J Glob Health. 2017;7:010902.

3 Sacks E, Freeman P, Sakyi K, Jennings M, Rassekh B, Gupta S, et al. Comprehensive review of the evidence regarding the effectiveness of community-based primary health care in improving maternal, neonatal and child health: 3. neonatal health findings. J Glob Health. 2017;7:010902.

4 Freeman P, Schleiff M, Sacks E, Rassekh B, Gupta S, Perry H. Comprehensive review of the evidence regarding the effectiveness of community-based primary health care in improving maternal, neonatal and child health: 4. child health findings. J Glob Health. 2017;7:010904.

5 Schleiff M, Kumapley R, Freeman P, Gupta S, Rassekh B, Perry H. Comprehensive review of the evidence regarding the effectiveness of community-based primary health care in improving maternal, neonatal and child health: 5. equity effects. J Glob Health. 2017;7:010905.

6 Perry H, Rassekh B, Gupta S, Freeman P. Comprehensive review of the evidence regarding the effectiveness of community-based primary health care in improving maternal, neonatal and child health: 6. strategies used by effective projects. J Glob Health. 2017;7:010906.

7 Perry H, Rassekh B, Gupta S, Freeman P. Comprehensive review of the evidence regarding the effectiveness of community-based primary health care in improving maternal, neonatal and child health: 7. programs with evidence of long-term impact on mortality in children younger than five years of age. J Glob Health. 2017;7:010907.

8 Victora CG, Requejo JH, Barros AJ, Berman P, Bhutta Z, Boerma T, et al. Countdown to 2015: a decade of tracking progress for maternal, newborn, and child survival. Lancet. 2016;387:2049-59. Medline:26477328 doi:10.1016/S0140-6736(15)00519-X

9 UNICEF. Tracking Progress in Maternal, Newborn and Child Survival. The 2008 Report. 2008. Available: http://www.who.int/pmnch/Countdownto2015FINALREPORT-apr7.pdf. Accessed: 26 February 2017.

10 Perry H, Freeman P, Gupta S, Rassekh B. How Effective Is Community-based Primary Health Care in Improving the Health of Children? Summary Findings and Report to the Expert Review Panel: American Public Health Association; 2009. Available: http://www.coregroup.org/storage/documents/finalcbphcreport_july2009.pdf and http://aimdb.files.wordpress.com/2009/08/finalcbphcreporttoerp-7july2009.pdf. Accessed: 26 February 2017.

11 Perry H, Freeman P, Gupta S, Rassekh B. Building on the Current Evidence to Strengthen Community-Based Service Delivery Strategies for Promoting Child Survival. 2010. Available: http://www.mchip.net/sites/default/files/USAID%20CBPHC%20FINAL.pdf. Accessed: 26 February 2017.

12 Freeman P, Perry HB, Gupta SK, Rassekh B. Accelerating progress in achieving the millennium development goal for children through community-based approaches. Glob Public Health. 2012;7:400-19. Medline:19890758 doi:10.1080/17441690903330305

13 United Nations General Assembly. Universal Declaration of Human Rights. 1948. Available: http://www.ohchr.org/EN/UDHR/Documents/UDHR_Translations/eng. pdf. Accessed: 26 February 2017.

14 World Health Organization. UNICEF. Declaration of Alma-Ata: International Conference on Primary Health Care. 1978. Available: http://www.who.int/publications/ almaata_declaration_en.pdf. Accessed: 27 February 2017.

15 World Health Organization. UNICEF, editors. Declaration of Alma-Ata. International Conference on Primary Health Care, 6-12 September 1978; 1978; Alma-Ata, USSR. Geneva, Switzerland: World Health Organization; 1978.

16 UN. Sustainable Development Goals. 2015. Available: https://sustainabledevelopment. un.org/topics/sustainabledevelopmentgoals. Accessed: 26 April 2017.

17 Chan M, Lake A. Towards ending preventable child deaths. Lancet. 2012;379:2119-20. Medline:22682447 doi:10.1016/S0140-6736(12)60908-8

18 Glass RI, Guttmacher AE, Black RE. Ending preventable child death in a generation. JAMA. 2012;308:141-2. Medline:22695930 doi:10.1001/jama.2012.7357

19 USAID. Acting on the Call: Ending Preventable Child and Maternal Deaths: A Focus on Equity. 2016. Available: https://www.usaid.gov/sites/default/files/Final-AOTC-file-v2. pdf. Accessed: 26 April 2017.

20 World Health Organization. The Global Strategy for Women's, Children's and Adolescents' Health (2016-2030): Survive, Thrive, Transform. 2016. Available: http://www. who.int/pmnch/media/events/2015/gs_2016_30.pdf. Accessed: 26 April 2017.

21 Black R, Walker N, Laxminarayan R, Temmerman M. Reproductive, Maternal, Newborn, and Child Health: Key Messages of This Volume. In: Black R, Laxminarayan R, Temmerman M, Walker N, editors. Reproductive, Maternal, Newborn, and Child Health. Washington, DC: World Bank; 2016.

22 Black RE, Levin C, Walker N, Chou D, Liu L, Temmerman M, et al. Reproductive, maternal, newborn, and child health: key messages from Disease Control Priorities 3rd Edition. Lancet. 2016;388:2811-24.

23 Lassi ZS, Kumar R, Bhutta ZA. Community-based care to improve maternal, newborn, and child health. 2016. In: Disease Control Priorities: Reproductive, Maternal, Newborn, and Child Health, Third Edition. Washington, DC: World Bank. Available: https://openknowledge.worldbank.org/bitstream/handle/10986/23833/9781464803482. pdf?sequence=3&isAllowed=y. Accessed: 26 February 2017.

24 World Health Organization. Multiple micronutrient supplementation during pregnancy. 2017. Available: http://www.who.int/elena/titles/micronutrients_pregnancy/en/. Accessed: 27 February 2017.

25 Szwarcwald CL, Souza-Junior PR, Damacena GN. Socioeconomic inequalities in the use of outpatient services in Brazil according to health care need: evidence from the World Health Survey. BMC Health Serv Res. 2010;10:217. Medline:20653970 doi:10.1186/1472-6963-10-217

26 Malik SM, Ashraf N. Equity in the use of public services for mother and newborn child health care in Pakistan: a utilization incidence analysis. Int J Equity Health. 2016;15:120. Medline:27459961 doi:10.1186/s12939-016-0405-x

27 Baqui AH, El-Arifeen S, Darmstadt GL, Ahmed S, Williams EK, Seraji HR, et al. Effect of community-based newborn-care intervention package implemented through two service-delivery strategies in Sylhet district, Bangladesh: a cluster-randomised controlled trial. Lancet. 2008;371:1936-44. Medline:18539225 doi:10.1016/S0140-6736(08)60835-1

28 Bryce J, Victora CG. Ten methodological lessons from the multi-country evaluation of integrated Management of Childhood Illness. Health Policy Plan. 2005;20 Suppl 1:i94-105. Medline:16306075 doi:10.1093/heapol/czi056

29 Nyonator FK, Awoonor-Williams JK, Phillips JF, Jones TC, Miller RA. The Ghana community-based health planning and services initiative for scaling up service delivery innovation. Health Policy Plan. 2005;20:25-34. Medline:15689427 doi:10.1093/heapol/czi003

30 Krumholz AR, Stone AE, Dalaba MA, Phillips JF, Adongo PB. Factors facilitating and constraining the scaling up of an evidence-based strategy of community-based primary care: management perspectives from northern Ghana. Glob Public Health. 2015;10:366-78. Medline:25436901 doi:10.1080/17441692.2014.981831

31 Awoonor-Williams JK, Phillips JF, Bawah AA. Catalyzing the scale-up of community-based primary healthcare in a rural impoverished region of northern Ghana. Int J Health Plann Manage. 2016;31:e273-89. Medline:26189569 doi:10.1002/hpm.2304

32 Shea BJ, Grimshaw JM, Wells GA, Boers M, Andersson N, Hamel C, et al. Development of AMSTAR: a measurement tool to assess the methodological quality of systematic reviews. BMC Med Res Methodol. 2007;7:10. Medline:17302989 doi:10.1186/1471-2288-7-10

33 Rosato M, Laverack G, Grabman LH, Tripathy P, Nair N, Mwansambo C, et al. Community participation: lessons for maternal, newborn, and child health. Lancet. 2008;372:962-71. Medline:18790319 doi:10.1016/S0140-6736(08)61406-3

34 Taylor CE. What would Jim Grant say now? Lancet. 2010;375:1236-7. Medline:20382313 doi:10.1016/S0140-6736(10)60449-7

35 Perry HB, Zulliger R, Rogers MM. Community Health Workers in low-, middle-, and high-income countries: an overview of their history, recent evolution, and current effectiveness. Annu Rev Public Health. 2014;35:399-421. Medline:24387091 doi:10.1146/annurev-publhealth-032013-182354

36 Hannay J, Heroux J. Community Health Workers and a Culture of Health: Lessons from U.S. and Global Models - A Learning Report. 2016. Available: http://www.rwjf.org/en/library/research/2016/08/community-health-workers-and-a-culture-of-health-lessons-from-u.html. Accessed: 27 February 2017.

37 El Arifeen S, Christou A, Reichenbach L, Osman FA, Azad K, Islam KS, et al. Community-based approaches and partnerships: innovations in health-service delivery in Bangladesh. Lancet. 2013;382:2012-26. Medline:24268607 doi:10.1016/S0140-6736(13)62149-2

38 Perry H, Scott K, Javadi D, Gergen J, Shelley K, Crigler L, et al. Case Studies of Large-Scale Community Health Worker Programs: Examples from Afghanistan, Bangladesh, Brazil, Ethiopia, India, Indonesia, Iran, Nepal, Niger, Pakistan, Rwanda, Zambia, and Zimbabwe. 2017. Washington, DC: USAID/MCSP. Available: http://www.mcsprogram.org/wp-content/uploads/2017/01/CHW-CaseStudies-Globes.pdf. Accessed: 26 February 2017.

39 Bang AT, Bang RA, Reddy HM. Home-based neonatal care: summary and applications of the field trial in rural Gadchiroli, India (1993 to 2003). J Perinatol. 2005;25 Suppl 1:S108-22. Medline:15791272 doi:10.1038/sj.jp.7211278

40 Taylor C, Parker R, DongLu D. China's model counties: Going to scale with health care. In: Taylor-Ide D, Taylor CE, editors. Just and Lasting Change: When Communities Own Their Futures. Baltimore and London: Johns Hopkins University Press; 2002. p. 284-95.

41 Taylor-Ide D, Taylor C. How to go to scale. In: Taylor-Ide D, Taylor CE, editors. Just and Lasting Change: When Communities Own Their Futures. Baltimore and London: Johns Hopkins University Press; 2002.

42 Arole M, Arole R. Jamkhed, India: The Evolution of a World Training Center. In: Taylor-Ide D, Taylor C, editors. Just and Lasting Change: When Communities Own Their Futures. Baltimore: Johns Hopkins University Press; 2002.

43 Paredes P, Taylor CE. Peru: Communities and Government Learning to Work Together. In: Taylor-Ide D, Taylor CE, editors. Just and Lasting Change: When Communities Own Their Futures. Baltimore and London: Johns Hopkins University Press; 2002.

44 Chowdhury AMR, Cash RA. A Simple Solution: Teaching Millions to Treat Diarrhoea at Home. Dhaka, Bangladesh: University Press Limited; 1996.

45 El-Saharty S, Janovsky K, Siadat B, Schleimann F. Seven Case Studies. In: Peters D, El-Saharty S, Siadat B, Janovsky K, Vujicic M, editors. Improving Health Service Delivery in Developing Countries: From Evidence to Action. Washington, DC: The World Bank; 2009.

46 Grant JP. Reaching the unreached: a miracle in the making. Asia Pac J Public Health. 1991;5:154-62. Medline:1818613 doi:10.1177/101053959100500209

47 Mahler H. Address to the 61st World Health Assembly. 2008. Available: http://www.who.int/mediacentre/events/2008/wha61/hafdan_mahler_speech/en/. Accessed: 26 February 2017.

48 United Nations. Sustainable Development Goals. 2015. Available: https://sustainabledevelopment.un.org/topics/sustainabledevelopmentgoals. Accessed: 26 February 2017.

49 Prata N, Vahidnia F, Potts M, Dries-Daffner I. Revisiting community-based distribution programs: are they still needed? Contraception. 2005;72:402-7. Medline:16307960 doi:10.1016/j.contraception.2005.06.059

50 Farmer P, Leandre F, Mukherjee JS, Claude M, Nevil P, Smith-Fawzi MC, et al. Community-based approaches to HIV treatment in resource-poor settings. Lancet. 2001;358:404-9. Medline:11502340 doi:10.1016/S0140-6736(01)05550-7

51 Chowdhury AM, Chowdhury S, Islam MN, Islam A, Vaughan JP. Control of tuberculosis by community health workers in Bangladesh. Lancet. 1997;350:169-72. Medline:9250184 doi:10.1016/S0140-6736(96)11311-8

52 Kidane G, Morrow RH. Teaching mothers to provide home treatment of malaria in Tigray, Ethiopia: a randomised trial. Lancet. 2000;356:550-5. Medline:10950232 doi:10.1016/S0140-6736(00)02580-0

53 Neupane D, Kallestrup P, McLachlan CS, Perry H. Community health workers for non-communicable diseases. Lancet Glob Health. 2014;2:e567. Medline:25304630 doi:10.1016/S2214-109X(14)70303-1

Acknowledgement: originally published as: Robert E Black, Carl E Taylor, Shobha Arole, Abhay Bang, Zulfiqar A Bhutta, A Mushtaque R Chowdhury, Betty R Kirkwood, Nazo Kureshy, Claudio F Lanata, James F Phillips, Mary Taylor, Cesar G Victora, Zonghan Zhu, Henry B Perry: Comprehensive review of the evidence regarding the effectiveness of Community–Based Primary Health Care in improving maternal, neonatal and child health: 8. summary and recommendations of the Expert Panel. Reprinted with permission from Edinburgh University Global Health Society under Creative Commons Attribution Licence (Journal of Global Health 2017; 010908).

Appendix 1.

Links to online supplementary materials.

Online supplementary material to Chapter 1:
http://jogh.org/documents/issue201701/jogh-07-010901-s001.pdf

Online supplementary material to Chapter 2:
http://jogh.org/documents/issue201701/jogh-07-010902-s001.pdf

Online supplementary material to Chapter 3:
http://jogh.org/documents/issue201701/jogh-07-010903-s001.pdf

Online supplementary material to Chapter 4:
http://jogh.org/documents/issue201701/jogh-07-010904-s001.pdf

Online supplementary material to Chapter 5:
http://jogh.org/documents/issue201701/jogh-07-010905-s001.pdf

Online supplementary material to Chapter 8:
http://jogh.org/documents/issue201701/jogh-07-010908-s001.pdf